Marketing Techniques
for
PHYSICAL THERAPISTS

Aspen Series in Physical Therapy
Carole B. Lewis, Series Editor

Marketing Techniques for PHYSICAL THERAPISTS

Kathryn Schaefer, PT, MPA
President
Physical Therapy Health Center
Arlington, Virginia

AN ASPEN PUBLICATION®
Aspen Publishers, Inc.
Gaithersburg, Maryland
1991

Library of Congress Cataloging-in-Publication Data

Schaefer, Kathryn.
Marketing techniques for physical therapists / Kathryn Schaefer.
p. cm. — (Aspen series in physical therapy)
Includes bibliographical references and index.
ISBN: 0-8342-0208-5
1. Physical therapy services—Marketing—Handbooks, manuals, etc. I. Title. II.
Series.
[DNLM: 1. Marketing of Health Services—methods—handbooks.
2. Physical Therapy—handbooks. WB 39 S294m]
RM713.S33 1991
362.1'78—dc20
DNLM/DLC
for Library of Congress
90-14570
CIP

Editorial Services: Ruth Bloom

Library of Congress Catalog Card Number: 90-14570
ISBN: 0-8342-0208-5

Printed in the United States of America

1 2 3 4 5

This book is dedicated
to my father,
Fred Schaefer,
who prepared me for life
with his intelligence, curiosity,
love, dedication to excellence,
and above all, his sense of humor.

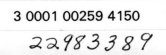

Table of Contents

Preface

Medical marketing is a young field. It has only been legal and considered professionally ethical to advertise health care since 1977, when the U.S. Supreme Court allowed professional advertising.[1] Prior to 1978, some hospitals had a small, usually one-person public relations department, but its functions were often limited to publishing an in-house newsletter, arranging occasional press interviews, developing and displaying patient education brochures, and organizing the annual hospital health fair.

Today, there is almost nothing written on this small and very specialized aspect of health care. The *Journal of Marketing* published one of the earliest medical marketing articles, which was written in 1971,[2] but a computerized literature search at the Library of Congress performed in June of 1989 revealed only thirty books printed on the subject. Additionally, almost all the medical marketing literature published to date addresses marketing for hospitals, health maintenance organizations, preferred provider organizations, and physicians. Articles and books on marketing allied health services are rare, and literature on marketing physical therapy is rarer still. Thus, the information compiled in this book is derived primarily from the medical marketing and general marketing literature combined with the author's marketing experiences in physical therapy in hospital settings and in private practice settings.

The intent of this book is to create a readable and easy-to-use text on marketing for the physical therapy clinician and manager. It is the author's belief that marketing physical therapy can be easy and fun. Furthermore, it is a natural extension and necessary adjunct to the way that we physical therapists currently manage our services.

NOTES

1. L. Sachs, *Do-It-Yourself Marketing for the Professional Practice* (Englewood Cliffs, N.J.: Prentice-Hall, Inc., 1986), xii.
2. P.D. Cooper, *Health Care Marketing Issues and Trends*, 2nd ed. (Gaithersburg, Md.: Aspen Publishers, Inc., 1985), 13.

Introduction

Physical therapists do not need expertise in marketing to market themselves, their clinics, and the profession effectively. Physical therapists do need a marketing text designed as a "cookbook" to help solve marketing problems with minimal effort and maximal results. This book was written with that premise in mind.

WHY MARKET?

In 1983, the Private Practice Section of the American Physical Therapy Association (APTA) hired a public relations firm to determine the image of physical therapy in the eye of the U.S. public. They found that the average U.S. citizen did not know what a physical therapist is and was unaware of the benefits of physical therapy. They reported that physical therapists did not have a strongly negative image—they essentially had no image at all. They told the APTA that a public relations firm does not consider this bad news, for it is easier to create a positive image out of no image than to reverse a negative image.

When this report was released, most physical therapists could identify with the results. We have all had frequent encounters with patients or new friends who either had the wrong impression of physical therapy or were frankly ignorant that the profession existed. Recently, for example, I was flying to a physical therapy seminar, and the person sitting next to me said, "You're a physical therapist? I could use a massage." I would love to have a dollar for every time someone has made that comment to me. I would gladly pay a dollar each time someone asked me an intelligent question about an exercise prescription or a biomechanical assessment.

I am sure that all physical therapists and physical therapy students have a story to tell about how they had to explain physical therapy and its benefits to family, friends, and even patients. Chances are that even the person who understood the role of the therapist in treating sports injuries had no idea about pediatric physical therapy or the role that physical therapists play in stroke rehabilitation or spinal cord injury. As a profession, physical therapy has a long way to go in educating the public about the profession, its services, and ways to obtain access to those services.

On a national level, the APTA and the Private Practice Section continue to use a public relations firm to promote physical therapy through features in national magazines, newspapers, television, and radio. Topics that have been publicized by the media nationwide include snowshoveling tips, briefcase elbow, tips for the couch potato, the prevention of falls in the elderly, and tips for the prevention of running injuries. The purpose of this media exposure is to position physical therapy as the unique health care specialty that it is and to present physical therapists as educated, knowledgeable professionals whom the public can trust.

The APTA and a public relations firm cannot change public opinion alone, however. At the local level, physical therapists can use this book to promote individual clinics, specialties, and themselves. The purpose of proper marketing is to educate the public about available services and to develop appropriate services to meet the physical therapy needs of the community.

Building a positive word-of-mouth reputation is the goal of all the marketing strategies presented in this book. Satisfied clients will return to the same clinic if they need further care and will recommend the clinic to their family and friends. Marketing studies show that one of the most important influences in a consumer's choice of a health care provider is a recommendation from a personal acquaintance. When reading and using this book, physical therapists should remember that the goals of market research, image development, internal marketing, public relations, advertising, and planning are to educate consumers about the benefits of physical therapy and to create satisfied clients who will promote the profession and its practitioners.

USE OF THIS BOOK

Professional physical therapists may not have the time, energy, or desire to study marketing in depth, but they may need to build their service through marketing activities. This book is intended to meet this need. It provides a marketing philosophy, as well as basic practical advice in marketing and promoting the physical therapy profession and physical therapy clinics.

Some physical therapists may read this book from start to finish for a comprehensive overview of marketing physical therapy. The book is designed primarily as a reference text, however, to provide a step-by-step guide to specific marketing activities, such as designing a brochure, creating a newsletter, preparing a speech, or developing an annual marketing plan. It describes what marketing for physical therapy is, why it is a vital part of the administrative process, and how marketing strategies can be easily applied to an individual practice setting.

This handbook is designed for physical therapists in all settings, including hospitals, nursing homes, home care, industry, and private practices, as well as for the physical therapy student who is about to enter a competitive health care market and, therefore, would benefit from a marketing orientation toward the profession of physical therapy.

MARKETING SKILLS OF PHYSICAL THERAPISTS

Effective management is primarily organized common sense and an ability to motivate people. These skills are similar to those needed in the day-to-day practice of a physical therapist. The keys to effective management are comprehensive and creative planning and evaluation. Marketing is a management process.

Effective marketing management boils down to four skills common to physical therapists. In our student training, we learn the skills of patient evaluation, problem solving, goal setting, and program planning. These skills are also taught to marketing students. Just as a physical therapist would not use a treatment tool such as ultrasound without first evaluating the patient's symptoms, designing a comprehensive treatment plan, and setting goals, a professional marketer would not consider creating a marketing tool such as a brochure without first evaluating the organization's needs, how it fits into the strategic marketing plan, and what marketing goals it will help to achieve. The processes of evaluation, planning, and goal setting are similar for both physical therapists and marketers.

The difference lies in the techniques. This book describes those marketing techniques that a physical therapist in almost any clinic setting, with even a small marketing budget, can readily perform. Incorporating these marketing techniques into a clinic's strategic plan and the practice of everyday management will enhance customer satisfaction, referral source satisfaction, and employee satisfaction. With proper marketing an organization is driven by its customers' needs; as a result, every employee understands and works toward the common goal. Success naturally follows.

When an organization's marketing needs are beyond the abilities of its staff, the choices for filling these needs are many. A graphic artist may be hired to design a logo, a market research firm may be hired to perform a needs analysis for placement of a satellite clinic in a neighboring community, or a full- or part-time marketing consultant may be hired to manage clinic growth and customer satisfaction. This book will help therapists determine when and how to use professional marketing assistance so that they can target their marketing efforts and dollars most effectively. The book's basic premise, however, is that many physical therapy clinics simply do not have the budget to seek outside expertise. When therapists understand basic marketing principles, they can design marketing strategies and tools for their organization. They can incorporate marketing at low cost and minimal personnel effort, using this book as a guide. Physical therapists already have most of the skills; this book provides the techniques for their application.

chapter 1

Marketing Theory

Health care marketing is the communication that occurs between the health care professional or organization and the health care consumer. It fills the gap between simply providing good services and making them accessible and available. Through marketing, the public learns when to seek medical care, how to recognize good care, and where to go for good medical care.

In order to use marketing techniques efficiently and economically, health care professionals and organizations must learn to identify the most appropriate target audience for information about their services. They must divide consumers into those who are more likely and those who are less likely to use the service, based on demographic characteristics and the product actually offered. This allows effective use of resources in the marketing effort. It is also necessary to determine how best to communicate the message about the services offered, based on the wants and needs of the consumer. This communication can be in writing—through brochures, newsletters, stationery, sales letters, and advertising. It can be in person—through sales calls, personal selling, and actual client interactions at the point of sale (e.g., before, during, and after treatment). The media can assist in communicating the health care provider's message through public service announcements, interviews, articles, and advertising. Marketing is a communication discipline that has much to offer the heath care provider who wishes to understand the wants and needs of the consumer and, as a result of this understanding, to create and enhance the services offered.

DEVELOPMENT OF THE MARKETING APPROACH

The focus of health care marketing is consumer satisfaction combined with professional competence and communication.[1] Marketing requires a close examination of the questions: Is the health care provider really giving patients what they want and need? If not, how can the provider meet consumer needs with services and then tell consumers about it? The marketing approach has evolved over time from two other approaches that organizations can take to communicate with the consumer about their products or services. They are the service approach and the selling approach.[2]

Service Approach

The foundation of the service approach is the theory that the consumer will purchase good services and facilities without marketing efforts.[3] Small-town physicians who hang a shingle out and wait for business to come in their door have adopted the service approach, for example. They assume that, as people in the community use their services, the services will speak for themselves and will be their marketing message. These physicians believe that any other type of promotion is unnecessary; they assume that their patients will know when to call for help and what the quality of their services is.

Over the years, many companies have successfully subscribed to Ralph Waldo Emerson's principle that, if a man can make a better mousetrap, the world will beat a path to his door. It is still true that no amount of aggressive marketing can take the place of a quality product that a consumer group wants and needs. Very little advertising was needed to promote the videocassette recorder (VCR) that was introduced in the late 1970s, for example, because it filled a consumer desire. Today, most households with a television set have at least one VCR as well. A physical therapy clinic can use the service concept to its advantage by recognizing the unique features of its services that match consumer desire. It can create a "better mousetrap" that will, to a certain extent, promote itself through word of mouth.

Organizations that use the service approach do not communicate, package, or promote a marketing message to consumers. The public learns of their service features, attributes, expertise, or technology strictly through word of mouth. Although this approach is extremely desirable because of the power of word-of-mouth promotions, the status attained through this concept may be short-lived. Health care continues to change dramatically in service provision and reimbursement structure; it is unwise to believe that providing good service is sufficient marketing. For example, a physical therapist may provide "the best mousetrap," but because of a government funding shift, may no longer receive reimbursement through government programs. Thus, the physical therapist's patients may go somewhere else where the services may not be as good, but are covered under these government programs.

The problem with the service approach to health care marketing is that the existence of health systems does not guarantee their survival. Physical therapists must not be so wrapped up in providing therapy as *they* think people need it and as *they* want to provide it that they forget to determine what the target public wants and needs. The most important part of marketing is determining the physical therapy needs of the community through market research and then communicating program benefits through public relations and advertising efforts. Because the service approach omits research and promotion, it falls short of a comprehensive marketing approach focused on complete customer satisfaction.[4]

The service approach worked well for marketing professional services several decades ago in small towns where no one was a stranger, and competition was minimal. Times have changed, however. Towns are now cities; many people do not know their neighbors; and competition in health care is rampant. The consumer is confused about what type of health insurance to buy and how to choose among various health care providers. Although programs that provide a quality product can use word-of-mouth promotions as a vital part of the marketing mix, it is necessary to go beyond the service approach to marketing in order to educate consumers about product benefits and to compete successfully in the marketplace. Table 1-1 lists the benefits and weaknesses of the service approach.

Selling Approach

Many advertisements in the media use a selling approach that assumes that the consumer will not purchase the product without an aggressive sales and promo-

Table 1-1 Comparison of Marketing Approaches

Approach	Benefits	Weaknesses
Service Approach: Good service sells itself.	Power of word-of-mouth promotions	Omission of market research Failure to take advantage of other promotional efforts
Selling Approach: Consumers will not buy product or service without hard-sell tactics.	Generation of sales that would otherwise not be made	Care essential to avoid deception Health care consumers' possible distrust and failure to respond to this approach
Marketing Approach: Organizations research consumer wants and needs; develop programs, products, and services based on the research; and communicate benefits offered through promotional efforts.	Consumer satisfaction Long-term success Promotions that reflect only benefits truly offered Consistency with the role of the health care professional	None

tional effort.[5] Mouthwash ads are good examples of the selling approach to marketing. The sellers assume that unless they market mouthwash aggressively—by linking it with the emotional appeal of attraction to the opposite sex, for instance—the consumer will not purchase the product. This aggressive sales approach is often the marketing technique of choice for used car sales and door-to-door encyclopedia sales as well.

In the selling approach, the sales pitch is often more important than the product or customer satisfaction. The sales pitch often consists of promises, giveaways, or emotional threats to stimulate sales: "Buy life insurance or your loved ones will be homeless and starving if you die." This hard-sell approach to marketing is the reason that many professionals still question the use of marketing in the health care field. Not only is it unethical to guarantee positive results or cures in health care, but also it may be illegal in some cases.

Unfortunately, some medical care marketing has already incorporated the worst aspects of the selling approach. A physician in a major metropolitan area took out a newspaper ad that stated, "Cure yourself of backache." Any physical therapist knows that this physician cannot possibly guarantee the cure promised in his ad. In health care, it is not always possible to keep results-oriented promises. This type of approach is designed to get new customers in the door, but the inability to provide the promised result inhibits follow-up marketing efforts.

It is sometimes easy for other types of deception to creep into hard-sell techniques. Although testimonials and endorsements are a very strong and useful form of advertising, care must be taken to avoid exaggeration or distortion of the benefits that can be expected from the service; pictorial representations must not mislead the consumer to expect qualitative outcomes that are not customary responses to treatment. The use of price reductions, discounts, and coupon advertising in health care also requires extreme caution to avoid deception. Prices may not be raised in order to reduce or discount them to a "customary" level; an aspect of service may not be called "free" if the charge for another aspect is raised to compensate for the "free" service. Hidden charges, such as finance charges, must be disclosed in the advertising.

Finally, creating benefits strictly for the purpose of selling a product is neither acceptable nor legal in medical marketing. In fact, promoting anything to anyone who has no need for it not only is unethical, but also will never generate satisfied customers—the ultimate goal of all marketing efforts.

The benefits and weaknesses of the selling approach are listed in Table 1-1.

Marketing Approach

By taking into account the critical importance of providing the best services possible as a part of the marketing picture, the marketing approach embraces the service approach. Services that tend to sell themselves through word of mouth are most legitimately marketed by the benefits that they actually offer to meet consumer need. The marketing approach first focuses on the wants, needs, and values of a target market in order to develop programs and services to meet those needs, wants, and values. This is followed by communication with the target market through various promotional efforts.[6] As marketing expert Peter Drucker stated, "The aim of marketing is to know and understand the consumer so well that the product or service fits him and sells itself."[7]

The attitudes behind the selling approach and the marketing approach are diametrically opposed. While marketing efforts in the selling approach are directed from the organization *at* the consumer, marketing efforts in the marketing approach are built on cooperation *with* the consumer to determine consumer needs. In the selling approach, for example, the organization examines the product or service that it has for sale and then designs promotions to make the consumer want to purchase that product or service. In contrast, an organization following the marketing approach first researches consumer wants and needs, then designs or modifies programs based on the research, and then informs consumers of the program benefits designed to meet their needs. The correct use and understanding of the marketing approach allows an organization to avoid the selling approach and still effectively generate new and repeat business. The marketing attitude is inherently designed for long-term success and customer satisfaction. The benefits of the marketing approach are listed in Table 1-1.

THREE CRITICAL CONCEPTS

All successful marketing efforts are based on an understanding of three critical marketing concepts:

1. target market
2. positioning for differential advantage
3. repetition and persistence

The target market is the specific segment of the population for whom programs and services are intended. Positioning for differential advantage involves placing a service uniquely in the mind of the target market by describing its major benefits, thus increasing consumer recognition and appropriate usage. Repetition and persistence are necessary because a target market requires multiple exposures to a marketing message before consumers understand and trust the benefits offered sufficiently to purchase the product or service.

Target Market

The population of the United States has various subsets with demographically similar characteristics. For example, the population can be divided by age (e.g., all those over 65 years of age), by sex (e.g., all females), by income (e.g., people who earn $25,000 to $30,000 per year), by location (e.g., all those living in the Virginia suburbs of Washington, D.C.), by purchasing habits (e.g., people who own BMWs), or by potential health care needs (e.g., weekend athletes). The target market of any organization is the specific subset of the population that may potentially want or need its services.

Historically, the primary target market for physical therapists has consisted of physicians. Because their profession is rapidly growing, physical therapists can now list consumers, insurance carriers, industry, and legislators as additional target markets. Consumers can be divided into submarkets, such as children, the elderly, and sports enthusiasts. Insurance companies are able to dictate the specific services that will be covered for reimbursement under their various policies and, therefore, need to be aware of the benefits of physical therapy. Big business and industry are target markets for those physical therapists who design and provide job site evaluation, work hardening, and back education programs. Legislators pass laws that define the scope of a physical therapy practice and, thus, are targets for marketing efforts. Even in states that have passed direct access legislation that allows consumers to seek physical therapy without a physician's referral, however, it is vital to maintain the physician–physical therapist referral relationship.

Choosing the target market is one of the first steps in any marketing effort. For physical therapists, the target market may be one of any number of subsets of specific groups within a category. Physicians, consumers, insurance carriers, and industry are the most common categories of target markets available to physical therapists. There are benefits to be derived and difficulties to be considered in targeting each potential group (Table 1-2). Although marketing efforts may begin with one of these groups as the primary target market, all four may be targeted once a comprehensive marketing program has been developed.

The Physician As the Target Market

Historically, the physician referral was the only way that a consumer could gain access to physical therapy services. Many clinics still rely exclusively on physician referrals for their patients. As the health care delivery system evolves, however, other methods of access are surfacing. For example, because the benefits of physical therapy are becoming more widely known, consumers are seeking services directly. More than half of the states now have legislation that permits consumer self-referral to physical therapy. Even in states with this legislation, however, physical therapy is a referral specialty, just as orthopedics, neurology,

Table 1-2 Benefits and Difficulties of Selected Target Markets

Target Market	Benefits	Difficulties
Physicians	Numerous referrals from influencing one referral source Targets easily identified by specialty Primary patient entry point to health care	Referral patterns often already established Can change referral patterns and go elsewhere
Consumers	Increased consumer choice in influencing their own health care decisions Improved consumer awareness of physical therapy benefits, which will increase demand	Expense In states without direct access laws, entry to the system still controlled by the physician Only one referral from influencing one consumer to use the service
Insurance carriers	Improved benefits for many referrals from influencing one insurance carrier Once one carrier changes policy, easier to convince others to do so	Expense Very little cost: benefit data available Great percentage of business affected by any change in policy
Industry	Profit in prevention programs Profit in pre-employment screening Profit in functional testing and work hardening programs	Often difficult to reach the decision maker Preconceived notions of proper way to manage health benefits expenses

and rheumatology are referral specialties. Therefore, although some patients seek out the specialist on their own through word of mouth or other methods, most are referred to the specialist by another practitioner.

The physician is no longer the only source of patient referrals for the physical therapist, but remains a valuable target market for many of the marketing efforts of the physical therapist. It is often cost-effective to recruit and retain a physician as a referral source, because one physician may refer numerous patients over a period of time. It is also easy to identify target physicians by their specialty and proximity to the clinic where the physical therapist practices. Physicians can also be targeted in most communities through the *Physician's Directory* published by the American Medical Association, a consumer's guide to local physicians, listings in the yellow pages, and hospital privilege lists, where physicians are listed alphabetically by name and also by specialty.

It is unwise for a physical therapist to rely too heavily on any one referral source for a major portion of his or her practice volume. There is always a possibility that a physician may send referrals elsewhere. This potential loss exists in hospital outpatient departments, as well as in private practice settings in which the physician either opens a self-owned physical therapy clinic or begins to refer patients to another clinic down the street for reasons beyond the physical therapist's control. A broad physician referral base is the most secure and stable marketing goal.

The Consumer As the Target Market

Demographically, a number of changes are occurring among U.S. health care consumers. They are becoming more conscious of health, fitness, and nutrition.[8] They are more likely to question a physician's diagnosis and treatment plan than ever before. They want more information about their symptoms, such as why they have them and what can be done about them. Almost every newspaper or magazine contains a health section with discussions of common ailments, self-diagnosis or treatment, and sources for the appropriate physician. Consumers are also more willing to accept responsibility for their health and even to make life style changes to improve their health, well-being, and quality of life. These demographic changes reveal a public ready and hungry for information about physical therapy services. In other words, consumers are ready as never before to receive marketing messages about these services.

Additionally, the national, state, and local marketing efforts of the American Physical Therapy Association (APTA), together with the efforts of individual clinics, are increasing consumer awareness of the benefits of physical therapy. As consumers learn how, when, and where to seek physical therapy, their potential importance as a target market increases.

Although consumers will increasingly become the target market of choice, there are several drawbacks to targeting this market. Marketing directly to consumers can be costly, because, unlike physicians, consumers may be completely unaware of the benefits of physical therapy; hence, more marketing exposure will be necessary. It is also harder to screen and select a consumer population segment that is likely to need physical therapy services. Some of the targeted population will be needlessly exposed to the message, at the therapist's expense. Furthermore, a number of marketing efforts may be required to bring a consumer to the decision to use the service, but all these efforts will result in only one referral.

The timing of marketing exposures to consumers is critical, as people require physical therapy only at certain points in their life cycles. A consumer who becomes aware of the service and the benefits offered through a successful marketing campaign, but does not need rehabilitation at the moment, may have forgotten the message two years later. Undertaking a consumer-oriented marketing plan involves long-term financial and strategic commitment. If such a plan is to be truly effective, the timing of the marketing messages must be fine-tuned to take into account the times in people's lives when they are most likely to need therapy. For example, therapists who offer sports physical therapy as one of their programs may find it useful to target the members of a local racquet club with a campaign on the treatment of tennis elbow or recurrent ankle sprains. Because they are actively participating in racquet sports, these people are more likely to need physical therapy at this time in their lives. They are also more likely to need rehabilitation services than is the adult population in general in any given community. Alternatively, a physical therapist may target the parents of high-school students who participate in athletics. In selecting either of these consumer groups, the therapist has timed the message to increase the likelihood of targeting a consumer group who may need physical therapy services.

The marketing techniques most commonly used in targeting the consumer are direct mail, listing in the yellow pages, public speaking, media interviews, and various forms of advertising. Each of these techniques may be costly in terms of dollars, time, and long-term commitment. Additionally, most of these techniques require paid, professional assistance. A consumer-oriented marketing campaign can be highly successful in promoting the image of physical therapists, instilling the benefits of their services, and increasing their visibility in the community, however.

The Insurance Carrier As the Target Market

Each insurance carrier establishes the rules and regulations that govern its reimbursement for physical therapy services. Many of those who currently create and implement these rules do not fully understand what physical therapy is and how it benefits patients. Therefore, they often develop guidelines that do not match patient needs and may not even be fiscally prudent for the insurance carrier.

It is essential to take a marketing approach toward educating major insurance carriers in order to ensure continued reimbursement for needed physical therapy services. Either the insurance committee of the state or district component of the APTA, or an individual physical therapist, can accomplish this task. The national APTA has literature and staff that can direct the therapist to helpful resources. For example, the APTA can provide information about such activities at the national level and can place a therapist in contact with those in other areas who are doing the same thing. Successful marketing with a private insurance carrier benefits all therapists in the area and can set positive precedents that can be used with other carriers. Therefore, if at all possible, it is advisable to unite resources in this marketing effort. Researching previously used strategies and position statements that have been successful, as well as those that have failed, can also be very helpful to therapists who are designing their own strategies.

The primary advantage in targeting an insurance carrier is that a large carrier's decision to establish generous coverage of physical therapy services brings about many referrals. It is important to remember, however, that many other providers are also heavily marketing the insurance carrier for the purpose of obtaining their share of the reimbursement dollar. With that knowledge in mind, physical therapists must educate insurance companies not only about the benefits of physical therapy, but also about the ways that physical therapy can help to reduce total insurance carrier expenses. Marketing techniques such as personal sales calls, marketing letters, telecommunications, brochures, and newsletters are appropriate educational tools.

Targeting insurance carriers is expensive in terms of time, effort, and dollars. Insurance carriers often have preconceived notions concerning the benefits and utilization of physical therapy that are difficult to change. These notions are best changed with data that substantiate the savings available to the insurance carrier through improvements in physical therapy benefits. Unfortunately, there are very few hard data to prove this point; the data that do exist can be obtained from the APTA, however. As competition for the health care dollar continues to grow, it becomes imperative that those in the physical therapy profession establish and maintain a significant voice in the halls of insurance carriers. Otherwise, the benefits available to patients in need may shrink year by year.

When selecting insurance carriers to target, a physical therapist should begin by studying the gross receipts (e.g., 1099 tax forms) from the last three to five years by insurance carrier. Ask your accountant to show you the end of the year 1099 tax forms that list your gross revenues per year for each carrier. A close study of the highest volume carriers may reveal any trends. A carrier whose referrals have been making up a steadily increasing percentage of the physical therapist's practice over the last several years is an obvious carrier to target. If a carrier has referred a high volume of patients for several years and the number of referrals suddenly declines, it is wise to investigate the cause of the change and to determine whether it can be remedied. At one clinic, referrals from the carrier that had sent the most patients for five years suddenly dropped off significantly in the first two months of 1989. Investigation revealed that the carrier had more than doubled its monthly premium in January. The major employer in the community had passed much of the increase on to the employee in the form of a co-payment, thus making the cost of remaining with this carrier prohibitive for many employees. The marketing/business decision was to seek the business of other carriers, as the premium co-payment was beyond the therapist's control.

Private carriers no longer offer the only type of health care insurance. Managed care is newer, but definitely established.[9] Managed care was developed in an attempt to reduce health care costs while maintaining the quality of the services provided. It includes all prepayment types of health insurance, such as health maintenance organizations (HMOs), preferred provider organizations (PPOs), and employer self-insurance. There is an advantage to targeting these groups in that contracts ensure payments for services; however, payments are likely to be at a reduced rate. Physical therapists must be sure that these reduced fees will cover their costs and maintain sufficient profit. Furthermore, because contracts come up for renewal periodically, it may be risky to rely solely or primarily on a managed care contract for referrals.

Industry As the Target Market

Industrial executives are acutely aware of their companies' rapidly increasing health insurance premiums and workers' compensation costs for employees injured on the job. Thus, many of the larger employers are moving toward self-insurance, as well as toward preventive health education and rehabilitation programs with proved track records for success. Because the physical therapist is uniquely positioned with the skills and expertise needed to institute these programs, marketing injury prevention programs, back education schools, pre-employment physical screening, postinjury rehabilitation programs, and work hardening programs can be extremely successful in this target market.

As large employers become more directly involved in defining and paying for the health benefits of their employees, they want information and programs designed to prevent large health care bills. These same industrial employers are concerned about the pre-employment fitness levels of job applicants. The cost to employers of on-the-job injuries through workers' compensation continues to rise, and employers want to hire workers who appear to be at low risk for injury. With their ability to perform pre-employment screening, physical therapists can help to determine each prospective employee's risk of injury.

Physical therapists can also offer objective testing of workers who have been injured to determine the level of disability and the activities that these workers can and cannot perform. If testing reveals weaknesses, a physical therapist can institute work hardening programs to strengthen the specific muscle groups that the employee needs on the job, thus allowing him or her to return to work. These physical therapy benefits can be successfully marketed to industrial executives as an objective method of minimizing costs.

Those who understand the benefits of physical therapy intervention in business find it difficult to believe that physical therapy programs are not more common in this market. Change takes time, however, and it is often difficult to get an appointment with the decision makers in industry to convince them of the benefits of physical therapy services. Additionally, many industrial executives still carry some preconceived notions about the management of health benefits expenses. Some are continuing to pay the ever increasing premiums of private health insurance without investigating cost containment measures. These industrial executives are not yet exploring creative risk management and incorporating it into union contracts. When this begins to happen, there will be a window of opportunity for physical therapists.

Positioning

In one year, the average consumer is exposed to approximately 200,000 advertising messages.[10] Consumers cannot possibly remember a message about physical therapy unless the message is simple and states the benefits of physical therapy from their point of view, rather than from the therapist's point of view. Positioning is the process of defining the product or service from the viewpoint of the target market.[11]

Positioning requires the simplification of a physical therapy clinic's activities into two or three simple phrases. Effective positioning helps the target market remember what the clinic is, what services it provides, and how it stands out among the competition. This is very important in our communication-saturated society.

Determination of Positioning Strategy

To position services so that they are understandable and meaningful to the target market, it is necessary first to know the clinic. A clinic's position is defined in its mission statement. In this statement, the organization's business objectives are described in broad and nonspecific terms.[12] For example, a hospital's mission statement may say, "The goal of this hospital is to meet the general acute medical and surgical needs of the people living in the community with specialties in obstetrics/gynecology, orthopedics, and sports medicine; and to remain financially viable as a nonprofit organization." The mission statement of the physical therapy department in that hospital may say, "The goal of this department is to develop and manage a general physical therapy department with a special emphasis on providing a sports physical therapy program focusing on the most common injuries prevailing in the community; and to remain financially viable." A mission statement should be one to three sentences in length. It states briefly and concisely not only the organization's goals, but also a strategy to achieve these goals.

In the above hospital example, the mission statement should include a strategy statement such as, "Strategies to meet these goals are to:

1. Perform focused and ongoing consumer and community needs research
2. Provide staff with professional credentials and advanced training in obstetrics/gynecology, orthopedics and sports medicine that match consumer and community needs
3. Provide technology and space for programs and treatments in obstetrics/gynecology, orthopedics and sports medicine that match consumer and community needs
4. Communicate the availability and salient characteristics of these programs to the appropriate target markets through marketing techniques listed in the annually updated market plan
5. Perform a cost/benefit analysis of each strategy to be included in its presentation for managerial approval."

The second step in the positioning process is to assess the strengths and weaknesses of personnel skills, acquired technology, size and quality of clinic space, and its location in the community. Such an assessment may be performed by a single physical therapist, the clinic's management team, or the entire staff. The more people involved in this process, however, the more objective and accurate the analysis. Referral sources and patients can be asked to list the clinic's strengths and weaknesses from their perspective and to include their comments on the form (Exhibit 1-1). Exhibit 1-2 is a completed example from Metropolitan Physical Therapy, a fictitious outpatient private practice.

Once the mission statement has been reviewed and the clinic's current strengths and weaknesses have been assessed, it is essential to analyze the needs of the consumer target market. This analysis, carried out by means of such techniques as demographic studies, focus group meetings, surveys, and interviews, provides information that can prevent costly marketing errors. For example, the community assessment may reveal significant demographic changes. If studies show an influx of young parents and an exodus of the elderly, the long-term viability and growth potential of a geriatric specialty clinic may be questioned. It may be necessary to reduce clinic size, to move the clinic, or to retrain the staff to meet the changing needs of the people in the community. Each of these options is a viable positioning strategy, depending on the organization's best interests. Assessing the target market in advance of actually marketing focuses efforts on areas that will yield maximum returns.

Assessing community needs in relation to the physical therapy clinic's current assets and mission can often provide valuable insight into the optimal position for the clinic. If the community assessment indicates that the most common types of injuries in the community are (1) industrial work-related injuries, (2) weekend athletic injuries, and (3) school sports injuries, the sports rehabilitation programs can be positioned in the marketplace accordingly. Furthermore, the community assessment may reveal the best ways to accomplish the organization's mission. In the previous example of the sports physical therapy clinic, the hospital and departmental mission statements are congruent and co-beneficial. Reorienting the physical therapy department toward a greater emphasis on sports rehabilitation also advances the hospital in its mission to specialize in sports medicine.

The clinic's position should be stated in terms of the benefits derived by the target population. It is a common error to describe a product's benefits in terms that are more meaningful to the provider than they are to the consumer. The first inclination of many health care providers is to talk about the modalities that they offer, the degrees that they hold, and the equipment that they have. The consumer is primarily interested in the answers to certain other questions, however: What's in it for me? Will my pain go away? How much better will I function? Will I play the sport again? The provider's position must be stated in terms that indicate the *outcome* that the *patient* will obtain from purchasing the services.

Exhibit 1-1 Clinic Assessment Form

Staff Skills Strengths	Weaknesses	Technology Strengths	Weaknesses	Space Strengths	Weaknesses	Location Strengths	Weaknesses
1.	1.	1.	1.	1.	1.	1.	1.
2.	2.	2.	2.	2.	2.	2.	2.
3.	3.	3.	3.	3.	3.	3.	3.
4.	4.	4.	4.	4.	4.	4.	4.
5.	5.	5.	5.	5.	5.	5.	5.
6.	6.	6.	6.	6.	6.	6.	6.

Exhibit 1-2 Clinic Assessment Form As Completed by Metropolitan Physical Therapy

Staff Skills		*Technology*		*Space*		*Location*	
Strengths	*Weaknesses*	*Strengths*	*Weaknesses*	*Strengths*	*Weaknesses*	*Strengths*	*Weaknesses*
1. Strong training	1. Don't know how to delegate tasks	1. Isokinetic equipment	1. Biofeedback machine broken	1. Attractive reception and business area	1. Halls too small	1. Easy to access by public transportation	1. Congested traffic
2. Advanced orthopedic skills	2. Documentation	2. High- and low-volt electrical stimulation	2. No neuroprobe	2. Private individual treatment rooms	2. Gym too small	2. Accessible to many businesses	2. Expensive parking
3. Compassion	3. Pediatrics	3. Whirlpool	3. No electromyographic equipment skills	3. Modern	3. Need to replace some pictures	3. Medical building well-known in community	3. Slow elevators
4. Good teamwork	4. Neurological training	4. Motorized cervical and pelvic traction		4. Clean			
5. Highly experienced	5. No marketing experience	5. Nordic track					
6. Managerial training and experience		6. Ergonomic bicycle					

Methods of Positioning

Services can be positioned in terms of product line, quality features, cost differentiation, or attributes and benefits.

Product Line Positioning. In health care, product line positioning was popularized in the late 1980s by hospitals that wished to make the complex of their services more understandable to the public. For a hospital, marketing a product line usually means creating a package of services from a number of departments. For example, a sports medicine product line includes services from the orthopedic, radiology, physical therapy, nursing, and, possibly, dietary departments. Other typical hospital product lines are cardiac rehabilitation, obstetrics/gynecology, and plastic surgery.

The major benefit of product line marketing is that those in a certain segment of the population instantly identify with the marketing message.[13] As a result, they become curious about the service and want to learn how it may benefit them. In other words, the product line message has a greater chance of penetrating the advertising message clutter and creating an impression that will be remembered than do some other types of messages. For example, if the marketing message for the sports medicine product line is "Weekend athletes can prevent serious injuries," those who consider themselves weekend athletes will immediately say, "That's me," and will listen to the rest of the message for further information. Few people identify with a message about the professional and caring orthopedic department at XYZ Hospital, however. If those who receive the marketing message think that the message is for someone else, they will not remember it; a specific message will yield a specific result.

A major disadvantage to product line marketing in a large organization such as a hospital results from the departmental structure of hospitals. Product line marketing often disrupts or short-circuits loyalties, budgets, and power, and there may be some resistance to the implementation of this positioning method by the various involved parties, as well as a power struggle for decision making. These obstacles should be anticipated and managed accordingly. With this consideration, product line marketing can be a very viable and successful positioning strategy for a large organization.

Smaller organizations with less departmentalization, such as a private practice physical therapy clinic, are often well suited to product line marketing. The physical therapist who specializes in sports physical therapy, pediatrics, or neurological disorders should promote that specialization as a product line. Smaller organizations may also have a disadvantage, however, in that they may be unable to offer a comprehensive, multiprofessional (one-stop shopping) package. Many physical therapy clinics are overcoming this disadvantage by hiring or establishing linkages with other professionals, such as dietitians, social workers, and exercise physiologists. In this way, they can market a more comprehensive package.

If physical therapy is the only component of the product line, it may be advantageous to focus the marketing message on the personalized and non-bureaucratic service rendered. The message may emphasize that the client will not get lost in the shuffle of people or paperwork.

Quality Features Positioning. Services can also be positioned by their quality features. This method of positioning relies heavily on creating and establishing a specific positive image with the target market and the community. The Pepsi Co. Incorporated positions its product as the soft drink of choice for fun activities, for example; its marketing efforts show people enjoying themselves in various ways while they are drinking Pepsi. Nike Incorporated positions its athletic shoes with the quality feature "excellence." Its ads show a short story in which a major athlete or individual achieves excellence, such as by winning a race. The ad is the story; Nike flashes its name only at the end of the ad.

To choose quality features with which to position a physical therapy clinic, it is necessary first to determine the features that are important to the target markets. Each target market should be surveyed individually. Because their perceptions and expectations differ, the message must differ for each group. For example, a physician may be interested in frequent communication concerning the patient's medical status, while the patient may be more interested in individualized and personalized treatment.

The results of consumer focus group sessions concerning physician quality attributes can be extrapolated to physical therapists: "According to consumers, a high-quality physician has a pleasant manner, exhibits a caring attitude, and communicates well with patients and their families."[14] Therefore, in designing a positioning strategy based on quality features, all marketing efforts should present the image of clinic therapists as good communicators who have caring attitudes and a pleasant manner.

Cost Differentiation Positioning. Although the elasticity of costs has a relatively small margin for difference in the pricing of physical therapy services, high and low costs can still be differentiated for the purpose of positioning. In the health care arena, however, cost differentiation is a risky way to position services.[15] People associate low cost with low quality and vice versa. This is a fact that physical therapists must understand whether they discount their services or charge high prices. The quality of discounted services will be perceived as lower than that of higher priced services. The benefit of providing low-cost services is that they become accessible to more people. In order to maintain profitability, however, it may be necessary to increase volume, reduce technology, or reduce staff. If part of the organization's mission statement is to treat all those in need of services, regardless of ability to pay, keeping charges low may be essential.

High prices are considered compatible with high quality. If the mission statement mandates the highest quality specialty service, it may be necessary to charge a premium rate to cover the costs that the clinic incurs in obtaining the finest equipment, space, and personnel. The costs incurred by the consumer are not only monetary. For example, the time taken off work to obtain treatment is a cost. The patient may perceive the pain or effort associated with treatment as a cost. Not to be considered lightly, there are costs incurred in filing insurance forms and waiting for reimbursement.

Attributes Positioning. The attributes of a clinic that may be used for positioning include its location, waiting time, technology, technical skills of personnel, and specialties offered. In this positioning method, the community's physical therapy needs are evaluated and compared to the competition's strengths and weaknesses. By matching community needs with the clinic's strengths and the competitors' weaknesses, it is possible to determine the clinic's optimal positioning strategy based on its attributes. One private practice outpatient clinic surveyed referring physicians and found that they would use a clinic that scheduled their patients shortly after they were referred. All the competitors had a significant waiting list. As a result of this knowledge, the clinic adopted a policy of scheduling all referrals within twenty-four hours. This positioning strategy has been very successful in marketing and retaining the physician referral sources.

Practical Applications

Designing a marketing strategy to position services so that they are understandable and meaningful to target markets requires an awareness that no clinic or service can be all things to all people. The public knows that a clinic cannot excel in *all* areas of physical therapy. If therapists promote themselves as generalists, the target public will assume that they provide standard, acceptable care, but the public may not realize that physical therapy is a specialized service that offers a great variety of benefits. Furthermore, not all physicians are fully aware of the numerous ways in which physical therapy may benefit their patients. Therefore, marketing efforts are more believable and effective when the service is positioned strategically.

Physical therapists can learn a lesson from product marketing. Xerox Corporation positions itself as the "copier company," while International Business Machines (IBM) positions itself as a "computer company." These companies know that the consumer will not believe that one company can successfully produce all things for all people. Therefore, they have reduced advertising clutter for the consumer and made their messages memorable. As a result, the purchasing consumer can focus on the quality attributes of their many product lines. Once Xerox has sold or leased a copier and is servicing it, the company hopes that the satisfied customer will develop brand loyalty and buy other Xerox products, such as computers.

In learning from product positioning strategies, physical therapists can select their own positioning strategy. They can position by product line, by quality features, by cost, or by attributes and benefits, thereby making their marketing message memorable, understandable, and more likely to penetrate the advertising message clutter the public must sift through every day. Exhibit 1-3 summarizes the steps required in assessing a physical therapy clinic's position in the marketplace.

Exhibit 1-3 Assessment of a Physical Therapy Clinic's Strategic Position

Assess Your Clinic's Current Position

1. What is your organization's mission statement?

2. What are your organizational strengths and weaknesses?

3. What are the demographic needs of the community served by your clinic?

4. What is your clinic's positioning strategy based on your answers to questions 1-3?

5. What are the potential product lines your clinic can offer?

6. What are the quality features that your clinic offers?

7. What is your current pricing strategy?

   Low Cost _____
   Moderate Cost _____
   High Cost _____

8. What are the clinic attributes that your target market needs that you specifically offer?

Repetition and Persistence

After sending out an announcement concerning the availability of services and following up with a telephone call to a referral source, many physical therapists are surprised that patients do not pour into their clinic. Being persistent, however, they send out follow-up letters and meet with a number of potential referral sources. Again, they are surprised and dismayed that referrals do not come flooding into their office. Finally, after several months of constant marketing activities, the clinic receives a significant number of referrals. The referral sources have responded to a marketing principle called "the hierarchy of effects."[16]

The hierarchy of effects represents the nine steps that consumers (the target market) must go through before they purchase an item or service. It recognizes that, in order to be effective, advertising and public relations depend on continuity and repetition to change consumer behavior. Marketing strategies must be aimed at bringing the target market through these nine steps (Exhibit 1-4).

When consumers are unaware that a service exists (step 1), they will obviously do nothing. Therefore, the first step in any marketing program is an awareness campaign. The purpose of such a campaign is simply to establish the beginning recognition of the name and of the existence of the service in the community (step 2). Once the target market is aware of the service, marketing strategies should bring the target market to an understanding of the function of the service or product (step 3). While an awareness campaign simply puts the name and the service in front of the target audience, an understanding campaign focuses on service attributes, such as the caring attitude and professionalism of the staff. The next step is to develop a familiarity with the product among the target market (step 4). At this stage, the caring professionalism of the staff may be demonstrated

---

Exhibit 1-4 Hierarchy of Effects

Hierarchy Steps (Consumer Perception)	*Expected Results* (Consumer Action)
1. Unawareness	Nothing
2. Awareness	Not much
3. Understanding	Recognition
4. Familiarity	Increased recognition
5. Interest	Acceptance and/or queries
6. Decision	Action
7. Satisfaction	Continued action
8. Repeat use	Increased referrals
9. Recommendation	Word-of-mouth promotion

through various examples in order to promote the target market's interest in buying the service (step 5).

Purchasers go through all these steps, consciously or unconsciously, before they actually decide to use a service. Therefore, physicians who show interest in a physical therapy clinic have not necessarily decided to send patients there. An evident interest in the clinic by the target market must be followed up with additional marketing strategies in order to promote decision making from the target market (step 6). Marketing strategy at this stage should address specific questions that consumers may have before they are willing to use the service. For example, a particular physician may refer patients to the clinic only after learning that the clinic has a Cybex isokinetic exercise unit or schedules patients within twenty-four hours of referral.

Once consumers have used the service, it is important to ensure that they are satisfied with the service (step 7). Customer satisfaction promotes repeat use of the service (step 8) and, ultimately, recommendation (step 9). The goal of every marketing effort is to promote repeat use and recommendation, because word of mouth is the most powerful marketing tool available.[17]

In one clinic, the hierarchy of effects was used to promote a geriatric program. Because the target market was initially unaware that a geriatric program existed, the clinic began with an awareness campaign (step 2). This consisted of a personal letter to currently referring physician groups such as orthopedists, geriatricians, internists, and rheumatologists. The letter explained the program and included information about free evaluation and treatment for patients who entered the research study that was being conducted.

To increase their understanding of the program (step 3), follow-up telephone calls were made to these physicians. Questions concerning the initial letter were asked and feedback considered. The goal at this stage was to determine the degree of curiosity about the program rather than to obtain actual referrals. To follow up on this curiosity and to move the target market toward familiarity (step 4), the clinic staff developed a newsletter devoted to the geriatric program and sent it to all currently referring physicians and other physicians listed by specialty in the local *Physicians Directory*.

To increase interest (step 5), copies of the program's protocol were sent to the most curious of the referral sources for their critique and comments. The clinic staff met with the nine physicians who expressed an interest in helping improve their protocol and research methodology. Not only did this interaction improve the protocol, but also the physicians came to trust the therapists' professional expertise in general and their ability to conduct this research program in particular. All of the physicians decided to send patients to the program (step 6).

Because the therapists at the clinic understood the hierarchy of effects, they knew that their marketing efforts could not end with the first referral. Their service had to meet the expectations of their referral sources. To ensure consumer

Exhibit 1-5 Hierarchy of Effects: Case Example Summary

Hierarchy Steps	Marketing Strategy
Step 1 Unawareness	Strategy 1 Preparation of program
Step 2 Awareness	Strategy 2 Letter to referral source
Step 3 Understanding	Strategy 3 Telemarketing
Step 4 Familiarity	Strategy 4 Newsletter
Step 5 Interest	Strategy 5 Personalized program with program specifics
Step 6 Decision	Strategy 6 Personal sales call
Step 7 Satisfaction	Strategy 7 Internal marketing
Step 8 Repeat use	Strategy 8 Internal marketing/telecommunications
Step 9 Recommendation	Strategy 9 Direct mail/telecommunications

satisfaction (step 7), they treated patients with respect and professionalism from the moment they called the office, through every interaction with staff, and even when they paid their final bill. Each referring physician received typed evaluation reports and updates, as well as discharge summaries. Achieving and maintaining satisfaction was and is a core aspect of marketing efforts.

The clinic maintained its marketing efforts with the referring physicians through telephone calls concerning current patients, periodic newsletters, and personal visits. This continued exposure was designed to foster repeat use (step 8) and recommendation of the service to other physicians (step 9). After all, word-of-mouth promotions and recommendations are the ultimate goals of all marketing. The challenge is to offer a program that is so needed by the community and so well carried out that the target market itself promotes the program (Exhibit 1-5).

An understanding of the consumer purchasing psychology of the hierarchy of effects can significantly improve physical therapists' marketing strategy by reinforcing the importance of repetition and persistence in the marketing campaign. If marketing efforts are not resulting in referrals, the target market should be reassessed to determine if consumers may simply be psychologically in the earlier stages of the hierarchy, which precede a decision to use or purchase the service. Repeating the message through various marketing techniques or strategies should result in an effective marketing campaign.

NOTES

1. P. Kotler and R.N. Clarke, *Marketing for Health Care Organizations* (Englewood Cliffs, N.J.: Prentice-Hall, Inc., 1987), 41.

2. P. Kotler, *Marketing Management*, 5th ed. (Englewood Cliffs, N.J.: Prentice-Hall, Inc., 1984), 17–20.

3. Ibid.

4. Ibid., 20.

5. Ibid., 19.

6. Ibid., 20–28.

7. Peter F. Drucker, *Management: Tasks, Responsibilities, and Practices* (New York: Harper & Row, 1973), 64–65.

8. J.P. Davidson, *The Marketing Sourcebook for Small Business* (New York: John Wiley & Sons, 1989), 3–20.

9. J. Mathews, ed., *Practice Issues in Physical Therapy* (Thorofare, N.J.: Slack, Inc, 1989), 109–126.

10. A. Ries and J. Trout, *Positioning: The Battle for Your Mind* (New York: McGraw-Hill Book Co., 1989), 196.

11. S.W. Brown et al., *Promoting Your Medical Practice* (Oradell, N.J.: Medical Economics Books, 1989), 47.

12. Kotler, *Marketing Management*, 45.

13. Ries and Trout, *Positioning: The Battle for Your Mind*, 132.

14. D.C. Coddington and K.D. Moore, *Market-Driven Strategies in Health Care* (San Francisco: Jossey-Bass Inc., Pub., 1987), 86.

15. R.S. MacStravic, ''Professional and Personal Quality of Care in Health Care Delivery,'' *Health Marketing Quarterly* 5 (1987/88):52, 75–87.

16. J.R. Evans and B. Berman, *Essentials of Marketing* (New York: MacMillian Publishing Co., Inc., 1984), 299.

17. S. Brown and A. Morley, *Marketing Strategies for Physicians: A Guide to Practice Growth* (Oradell, N.J.: Medical Economics Company, Inc., 1986), 169–176.

chapter 2

Strategic Marketing Planning

PURPOSE OF PLANNING

An organization's managers must plan in order to recognize formally where the organization was yesterday, where it is today, and where it should be tomorrow. Planning provides structure and logic to the thought process of management. It confirms the organization's mission; takes into account the influences of the external environment; permits the identification of opportunities and difficulties in the marketplace; and creates goals, objectives, strategies, and evaluation measures to monitor performance. More specifically, it

- provides direction for marketing efforts
- provides a means to measure progress
- establishes a base for follow-up planning
- promotes organized thinking
- pinpoints strengths and weaknesses
- identifies competitive position
- sets proper priorities
- coordinates marketing strategies and tactics
- establishes a time frame for deadlines
- keeps the focus on results
- provides a working document
- permits meaningful program evaluation.

Planning is developing "a method for achieving an end."[1] It is essential to perform the planning process at least annually and to measure actual performance at least monthly.

Although the formal planning process is necessary for success, following the plan to the absolute letter can precipitate failure. Business operates in a changing environment, with changing customer needs, changing competitive forces, and a changing marketplace. A plan must be flexible enough to adapt to these changes as they occur, since they cannot all be foreseen during the planning process.

Planning is a major topic of business and marketing management literature. The primary common denominator among the planning processes described is the recognition of the importance of going through the planning process in order to ensure that the organization's activities are directed toward specific objectives, goals, and missions. It is all too easy for an organization, a department, or a division to be sidetracked from the organizational mission by the personal ambitions of individuals or by a task that appears too difficult. For example, the head of a physical therapy department in a hospital must maintain the hospital's mission and goals as a focus for planning rather than allow the focus to shift to departmental turf battles over who has the largest budget or biggest program. Similarly, the head of the department must not use the demands of day-to-day operations, supervision of employee performance, and customer complaints to justify a failure to work toward a goal that may seem difficult, such as obtaining greater visibility in the community. Performing the planning process regularly can help keep the organization on track and focused on its true mission.

COORDINATION WITH ORGANIZATION'S STRATEGIC PLAN

The marketing plan for physical therapy services must be designed in coordination with the organization's overall strategic plan. Each goal is derived from the mission statement and should clearly direct the organization toward its mission. Johnston and Lord, in their book *Your Private Practice "Planning and Organization"* state several advantages of goal setting:

- Yields reflection upon organizational purpose
- Identifies success
- Eases the decision process
- Increases personal confidence
- Saves time
- Provides framework for the organizational planning
- Provides a sense of rationality and order[2(p.4)]

The strategic plan contains four components that are essential to the marketing plan: the mission statement, the organizational goals, the fiscal goals, and the qualitative goals (Exhibit 2-1). Exhibit 2-2 shows how a fictitious physical ther-

Exhibit 2-1 Organizational Strategic Plan Form

<u>Strategic Plan</u>

1. <u>Mission Statement</u>:

   _____

   _____

2. <u>Organizational Growth Goals</u> (i.e., added programs, space, staff):

   _____

   _____

3. <u>Fiscal Goals</u> (i.e., percentage increase in gross revenue, profitability):

   _____

   _____

4. <u>Qualitative Goals</u> (i.e., enhancement of technology, image, personnel, specialties, customer relations):

   _____

   _____

Exhibit 2-2 Completed Organizational Strategic Plan Form

<u>Strategic Plan</u>

1. <u>Mission Statement</u>: To provide an outpatient medical environment conducive to the attainment of optimal musculoskeletal health and well-being that operates on the cutting edge of technological and clinical skills in the field of physical therapy and parallels community need in this field while maintaining profitability

2. <u>Organizational Growth Goals</u>:
   - Investigate a senior wellness product line
   - Investigate weekend athlete product line
   - Double office space
   - Increase professional and support staff

3. <u>Fiscal Goals</u>:
   - 75% increase in gross revenue
   - 10% increase in profitability

4. <u>Qualitative Goals</u>:
   - Purchase isokinetic equipment
   - Enhance community image
   - Evaluate personnel skills in each job description and provide educational opportunities to enhance skill level
   - Evaluate and enhance customer relations

apy private practice completed Exhibit 2-1. The goals listed in the example foster the accomplishment of the mission statement. Tying the growth, fiscal, and qualitative goals to the organization's mission ensures that all activities contribute to the mission and thus to the success of the organization.

MARKET RESEARCH

In order to put together a market plan, it is necessary to conduct market research. Kotler, one of the gurus of marketing, defined market research as "the systematic design, collection, analysis and reporting of data and findings relative to a specific marketing situation facing an organization."[3] Market research is the scientific arm of marketing. Therefore, it requires accuracy and objectivity, it must be unbiased, and the research tools must be carefully developed and used. Without market research, information about the community, the environment, and potential patients comes from intuition, hunches, and guesses. Although such factors can often suggest appropriate directions for market research and initial assumptions for further study, conclusions based on intuitive information are not scientifically valid and may be inaccurate.

Although market research can be expensive and time-consuming, gathering the data required to make good marketing decisions need not always be either. Physical therapists can do much of their own market research by tapping into known resources and by staying close to their customers.

Market research information can be gathered from numerous sources.

- physical therapy practitioners
- referral sources (e.g., physicians, health maintenance organizations [HMOs], preferred provider organizations [PPOs])
- local American Medical Association (AMA) and American Physical Therapy Association (APTA) chapters
- patients
- directors of community groups serving the target group
- community leaders
- health care institutions
- mayor/governor's office
- Census Bureau
- research health care data collection centers (e.g., Donnelly Marketing Information Services)

Other physical therapy practitioners who work in the community may have a great deal of information that they are willing to share. The local Chamber of Commerce is likely to have information concerning aging, economic, and business trends in the community. Referral sources and local leaders in the health care fields may also be able to provide information on the trends in the community. The opinions of current patients, directors of community groups that already serve the target groups (e.g., church leaders), and local elected officials (e.g., the mayor and city council members) are often valuable. There are also research health care data collection centers, such as the Donnelly Marketing Information Services, that collect and sell health care statistical data.

The purpose of much of the market research performed by large businesses is to stay close to the customer. As a general rule, the larger the business, the farther from the customer the decision makers. The lowest paid employees are frequently the people who actually interact with the customer and are most familiar with the customer's wants, needs, attitudes, perceptions, and beliefs about the product or service. This is as true for the Xerox Corporation as it is for Kaiser Permanente and the local community hospital.

It is much easier for small-business decision makers to stay close to the consumer, as they are often in direct, daily contact with the customer. Because of the nature of physical therapy, many physical therapists already have much of the customer information that they need to make expansion and programming decisions. Unless the opportunity is taken during the consumer interaction to ask specific opinion-generating questions, however, the information held by the physical therapist may be incomplete.

Data Collection

Information concerning the viability, potential, and opportunities for existing and new physical therapy clinics is readily accessible. It can be obtained through demographic analyses, focus group discussions, mail surveys, telephone surveys, consumer preference analyses, computer analyses, man-on-the-street interviews, and personal interviews. This information should be updated regularly to ensure the continued focus and accuracy of the marketing plan. A successful clinic generally reassesses this information at least annually in order to update services offered and stay ahead of the competition.

Demographic Analyses

Market research techniques include the study of changing demographic trends nationally and locally as they affect the physical therapy market. Regular demographic market analyses keep a business positioned to take advantage of environmental changes.

Age Analysis. Physical therapists should begin demographic analyses by determining aging trends, both nationally and locally. Nationally, the U.S. population is aging. There is now and will continue to be an ever increasing number of elderly people. Aging trends should also be studied in the local community to create a complete picture, as this population group is not increasing in all communities. A form such as that shown in Exhibit 2-3 can be used to record whether various age groups are increasing or decreasing nationally and locally.

The members of this growing consumer group are better educated, wealthier, and more discriminating than previous elderly populations were. Their physical therapy needs are different from those of younger adults because the physiological changes associated with aging slow the healing process. As the elderly in the United States increase, study of their health care needs is likely to indicate that they are a strong potential target market for physical therapy clinics.

Economic Analysis. As in an age analysis, it is helpful to track economic demographic characteristics on both the national and the local level. The national interest rate, average family income, cost of living increases, and stock market fluctuations indicate the financial mood of the country. This mood affects bank lending policies, investor risk potential, and consumer attitudes toward any co-payments that they may be required to make. Because local economic trends may differ from national trends, the average family income in the community should be compared to the national average. The local job market, as well as the industries and businesses that support the local economy, should be considered. Are these industries in the growth, plateau, or decline stage of the business life cycle? Are they moving into or out of the community? Economic factors locally and nationally affect the viability of a physical therapy clinic.

Community Resources

In performing market research, physical therapists should take into account every facility in the area that provides services even slightly similar to the planned

---

Exhibit 2-3 Record Form for Aging Trends

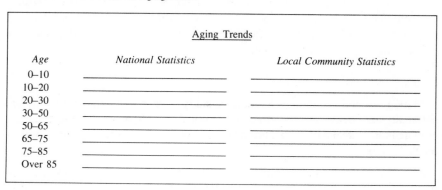

Age	National Statistics	Local Community Statistics
0–10		
10–20		
20–30		
30–50		
50–65		
65–75		
75–85		
Over 85		

Aging Trends

service. For example, a physical therapist who treats primarily sports injuries should list every facility in the community where people currently seek information on the management of sports injuries, including the public library, local health clubs, physicians of all specialty areas (e.g., internal medicine, orthopaedics, podiatry), other physical therapy clinics, chiropractors, and even sports call-in radio and television shows with health care professionals as hosts. It is essential to determine if these existing resources are currently meeting the total demand for services in the area or if some members of the community are traveling further to meet their sports rehabilitation needs. If these current resources are meeting the total demand, there is no room for another clinic. Even if the existing resources are currently managing the entire market share, however, there may be room for a facility that manages sports rehabilitation in a different way; it may be possible, by providing a unique service, to capture a percentage of the currently existing market and take consumers away from the competition.

Once existing resources in the community have been listed and analyzed, the next step is to determine whether there are any health care gaps, any physical therapy needs that are not currently being met. Potential gaps should be investigated in terms of:

- product line
- location
- service
- cost.

Physical therapy product lines that may not be available in the community include sports rehabilitation, pediatrics, obstetrics/gynecology, work hardening, pre-employment screening, geriatrics, pain management, and home care. If these product lines are available, they may not be accessible to all consumers because of a poor location; this is especially true for the outpatient physical therapy services, which often require several visits to a clinic in a week. Unfortunately, many health care facilities are still not as service-oriented as consumers would like. Large amounts of paperwork, long waiting times, and a lack of professionalism in existing organizations can create opportunities for new organizations. Charges may also cause a potential gap for a new competitor. A small, free-standing clinic can sometimes offer services for lower charges because its overhead expenses are lower. Large hospitals, for example, often require income-producing departments, such as a physical therapy department, to support the overhead expenses of other services, such as nursing, housekeeping, and dietary. These types of health care gaps may offer a marketing niche for an existing, expanding, or new physical therapy clinic.

It is also essential to assess the attitudes of the physicians in the community toward the existing services, including their receptivity to a new physical therapy clinic. Even in states that have enacted legislation to allow consumers direct access to physical therapy services, most referrals still come from physicians. Family practitioners and physicians who specialize in internal medicine may have been referring patients to other physician specialists and losing their patients to follow-up with those other physicians. They may be more than willing to send patients to an alternative or new physical therapy clinic.

In some communities, consumers are assertive and independent in decision making concerning their health care wants and needs, and they are interested in alternative health care resources. These community attitudes have a strong impact on the positioning and marketing of a physical therapy facility. Frequently, physical therapists find the community essentially unaware of the benefits of physical therapy and receptive to an awareness campaign.

Self-Assessment

The strengths and weaknesses of the physical therapy clinic as an organization and of the individual therapists who practice there must be examined. It is essential to be as objective as possible. After this self-assessment, the strengths and weaknesses can be matched with community needs in order to determine the viability of the particular program or proposed clinic.

The location of a proposed clinic is particularly important, as it relates to accessibility and image. It is essential to examine the availability of transportation to the clinic: How easy is it to get there by car, and how easy is it to park? Is public transportation available? Is the image of the neighborhood urban, business, or residential? How does the location affect the hours of operation? (See Exhibit 2-4 for data collection and background information areas.)

Focus Group Sessions

A focus group session is a meeting in which eight to twelve members of the target market brainstorm under the leadership of a moderator. The focus group

---

Exhibit 2-4 Data Collection—Background Information

- Demographics
  —Age
  —Economics
- Existing Resources
- Health Care Gaps
- Physician Attitude
- Community Attitude
- Self-Assessment
- Location

discuss their feelings, attitudes, and perceptions on a particular topic. Sessions usually last approximately one hour, and, although they are led by the moderator, they are meant to be free form. The purpose is to obtain in-depth information about the attitudes, opinions, and beliefs of the group rather than to obtain the hard numerical statistics of a survey. The focus group may generate information that can be used to design a survey, however.

Consumer reaction to various potential products or services may be valuable during the development and planning stage of a product. Comparative perceptions on existing providers and their services can also be elicited in a focus group. General attitudes and preferences concerning the importance of various service quality features, such as the helpfulness, caring, and knowledgeability of providers, and even the decor of facilities, can be elicited in focus groups. On the other hand, the focus group may simply discuss new ideas to improve market position and penetration may be the purpose. For example, the focus group may try to answer the question: Why do physicians refer patients to physical therapists? To answer that question, a professional moderator may lead eight to twelve physicians in a one-hour discussion of the overt and hidden attitudes, opinions, and beliefs about the reasons that physicians refer patients to physical therapy. Answers from a focus group such as this can help guide future physical therapy marketing efforts toward the goal of increased physician referrals.

The participants in a focus group are ordinarily paid. Currently, consumers generally receive approximately $50.00 for one hour of time, plus a meal. Physicians usually receive $100 to $150, plus a meal, for their participation.

A focus group can be a very effective information-gathering tool. It is wise to hire a professional focus group moderator, someone who is trained in developing focus group questions and guiding conversations in order to obtain the desired information objectively.

Surveys

Any target market, including physicians, patients, and potential patients, can be surveyed. Surveys can be performed by mail, by telephone, or in public places such as malls. Although it is preferable for surveys to be designed by professionals, many small businesses find this cost prohibitive and design their own. Following are a few simple guidelines in survey design:

- Keep the survey short, one side of one page if possible.
- Avoid requesting long written answers.
- Ask for answers on a scale.
  1. like, no opinion, dislike
  2. yes, no
  3. excellent, good, average, poor
  4. very important, somewhat important, not important

- Ask targeted questions that provide information useful to strategic planning and marketing.
- Provide space for additional comments at the end.
- Always enclose a self-addressed, stamped envelope to improve returns.

If the customer satisfaction surveys are designed in-house or are modeled after other surveys, they will be less expensive; however, they may not ask the right questions or generate the responses that are needed. Weaknesses of consumer surveys are possible low response rate and potential design bias.

Experts vary on the return rates required to permit valid conclusions, with the range being from 15 percent to 30 percent. Although surveys designed by non-marketing experts are probably biased, much useful information can be collected in this way. Exhibits 2-5 and 2-6 are surveys designed at one physical therapy clinic to track physician and patient attitudes over time. The physician survey is sent biannually, and the patient survey is given to all patients at the time of discharge.

If the results of a telephone survey are to be accurate, the telemarketers (i.e., the people conducting the survey) must ask the same questions in exactly the same way every time. In order to avoid the pitfalls of a survey, it is important to have several people review the survey questions to ensure that the questions are worded correctly and are not misleading, insensitive, or incomprehensible. In constructing the survey, the goals must be clearly stated during the planning stage so that no unnecessary questions are included and no necessary questions are excluded. For example, the questions in a survey of physicians to evaluate their satisfaction with physical therapy services would be very different from those in a survey to determine physician awareness of these services. Finally, it is essential to ensure that the sample population being surveyed accurately reflects the target population.

Interviews

Man-on-the-street interviews can be done best by a public relations firm. Such interviews are designed to elicit general information from people at a particular site. They can be videotaped and viewed later by those who commissioned the interviews. It is helpful to conduct man-on-the-street interviews before and after a general public awareness campaign in order to determine the effectiveness of the campaign.

Personal interviews with one or more members of a target market can elicit excellent research information. These interviews may be formal or informal. Informal interviews are conversations that occur by chance, as with patients who are leaving the clinic or with a physician who is in the hospital hallway or health club. Information obtained in this way should be recorded in a marketing file for future use and reference. Formal interviews are scheduled in advance and follow the procedures and format of sales calls.

Exhibit 2-5 Physician Survey

Because we value our relationship with you and wish to continue to provide your patients with the best possible physical therapy, we ask that you fill out the enclosed survey and return it to us in the enclosed self-addressed, stamped envelope.

	Yes	No
1. In general, I am satisfied with the services provided.	☐	☐
2. Reports are timely.	☐	☐
3. Reports provide sufficient information.	☐	☐
4. I am satisfied with the quality of physical therapy my patients receive.	☐	☐
5. My patients are satisfied with the quality.	☐	☐
6. My patients are satisfied with the facility and equipment.	☐	☐
7. I would send patients to you again.	☐	☐

8. Please number in order of preference the attributes you think are important in choosing a physical therapist.

Convenient hours   _____
No waiting   _____
Explanation of procedures to patients   _____
Convenient office location   _____
Education and training   _____
Experience   _____
Good personality   _____

9. Please list any complaints or problems you have experienced.

_____
_____
_____

10. Please list any complaints or problems your patients have experienced.

_____
_____
_____

11. Other comments:

_____
_____
_____

Thank you for entrusting your patients to our care. We look forward to providing a continuing and ever improving physical therapy service to your patients.
With kindest personal regards, we remain,

Computer Analysis

One form of market research that can easily be done in-house involves the clinic's computer. Monthly and annual statistics, such as patient age, diagnosis, referring physician, home address, and form of payment, may be charted. An examination of the trends thus revealed by the computer analysis can indicate the effectivensss of various marketing programs.

Exhibit 2-6 Patient Survey

Date _____
Name _____

Dear Patient:

Thank you for choosing our clinic. Your comments about the clinic are important to us. To assist us in our efforts to improve our services, please take a few minutes to answer the following questions. Thank you for your assistance.

1. Was this your first visit to our clinic? _____ yes _____ no
2. Were you aware of our clinic before your physician referred you here?
   _____ yes _____ no
   If yes, how did you hear of us? _____
3. Was this your first experience with physical therapy?
   _____ yes _____ no
4. Which features of our clinic influenced you to use our services?
   Please rate the following in importance to you.

	Very Important	Somewhat Important	Not Important
a) Location	_____	_____	_____
b) Cost	_____	_____	_____
c) All professional staff	_____	_____	_____
d) Doctor expressed preference	_____	_____	_____
e) Reputation in community	_____	_____	_____
f) Hours of service	_____	_____	_____

5. How long on the average did you have to wait in the reception area?
   Less than 5 min., _____ 5–15 min., _____ 15–30 min., _____ 30+ min _____
6. From your experience in our clinic, please rate the following:

	Excellent	Good	Average	Poor
a) Telephone	_____	_____	_____	_____
b) Parking facilities	_____	_____	_____	_____
c) Waiting area	_____	_____	_____	_____
d) Payment procedures	_____	_____	_____	_____
e) Cost	_____	_____	_____	_____

7. How well did the care you received meet your expectations?
   Exceeded expectations _____ Met my expectations _____
   Did not meet my expectations at all _____
   If you found any services lacking, what would you like to see included? _____
   _____

8. Did the receptionist:
   a) Greet you pleasantly _____ yes _____ no
   b) Handle payment efficiently _____ yes _____ no
   c) Seem to be (check all that apply)
      Competent _____ Concerned _____ Disrespectful _____
      Courteous _____ Inefficient _____ Unconcerned _____
      Other _____

Exhibit 2-6 continued

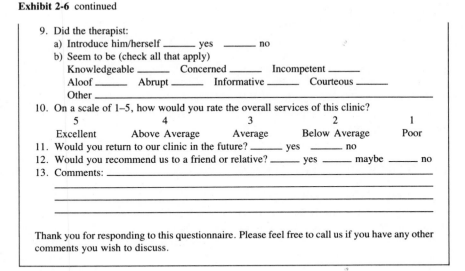

9. Did the therapist:
   a) Introduce him/herself _____ yes _____ no
   b) Seem to be (check all that apply)
      Knowledgeable _____ Concerned _____ Incompetent _____
      Aloof _____ Abrupt _____ Informative _____ Courteous _____
      Other _____
10. On a scale of 1–5, how would you rate the overall services of this clinic?

5	4	3	2	1
Excellent	Above Average	Average	Below Average	Poor

11. Would you return to our clinic in the future? _____ yes _____ no
12. Would you recommend us to a friend or relative? _____ yes _____ maybe _____ no
13. Comments: _____
    _____
    _____
    _____

Thank you for responding to this questionnaire. Please feel free to call us if you have any other comments you wish to discuss.

Research Budget

It is difficult to say how much of an organization's budget should be spent or is typically spent on market research. Large commercial companies in the U.S. budget between 0.01 percent and 3.5 percent of their sales to market research; approximately 50 percent of this amount goes to outside research firms that perform studies for the organizations.[4] These statistics do not readily apply to physical therapy clinics or even rehabilitation centers, because most are considered small businesses. The smaller the business, the smaller the percentage of the budget that is allotted for market research. It is unrealistic to believe that an individual physical therapist can afford all the objective scientific market research necessary to ensure that a product will meet consumer needs and will be designed and evaluated according to scientific principles.

Market research performed by consulting firms is costly. One focus group session can cost $2,000.[5] One consumer survey can cost more than $5,000. The information obtained through any one research activity is likely to answer only one or two questions about the market, however, necessitating multiple simultaneous studies. Furthermore, market research should be performed both before and after a product or service is introduced in order to determine its effectiveness and consumer attitudes, beliefs, and opinions.

The fact that most physical therapists' research budgets are small is not an excuse to avoid market research altogether. Small businesses can borrow many of the market research techniques used by large companies to improve decision making in program planning and service delivery. Focus group sessions, surveys, and personal interviews are all research methods that small businesses can use successfully to gather the information needed for sound business decisions. When research studies are designed and performed in-house by people not trained in marketing, caution must be employed in interpretation. The results may be flawed and biased. Simply recognizing the bias of this information can make it useful, however. Any assumptions made in creating the research tool should be listed, as well as the desired outcomes that may bias the research report. By taking possible biases into account, small businesses can take advantage of market research techniques that are otherwise far beyond their budget.

DEVELOPMENT OF THE MARKET PLAN

Once research has revealed the necessary information about the community, the environment, consumer need, and internal strengths and weaknesses, this information can be put to use in the market plan. Key staff members should be involved in this early phase of planning (Exhibit 2-7). They can help gather as much information as possible for the marketing program, determine the roles that each individual will play, and discuss the impact that the project will have on the various staff members. Involving staff members at this time creates an atmosphere of teamwork and avoids the impression that the marketer is the sole planner and implementor of the market plan. Participatory management breeds a supportive and enthusiastic staff.

This market plan is for internal planning purposes only. Other market plans may be designed with the goal of obtaining bank financing or interesting venture capitalists. This is not the purpose of the market plan, however. The purpose of the market plan is to organize marketing tactics into a clear strategy that propels the organization's mission and goals forward.

There are twelve steps in the market plan (Exhibit 2-8).

1. Describe the internal business environment, which consists of the aspects of the business that are already in place. This includes both strengths (e.g., highly trained personnel, an attractive facility, and well thought out policies and procedures) and weaknesses (e.g., insufficient personnel, space shortage, and policies that aren't followed).

Exhibit 2-7 Benefits of Involving Staff in Market Plan Design

- Assist data collection
- Discuss roles and impact
- Create teamwork and support

Exhibit 2-8 Market Plan

1. Describe the internal business environment.

   Strengths   *Weaknesses*

   _____   _____
   _____   _____
   _____   _____

2. Describe the external business environment.

   Opportunities   *Threats*

   _____   _____
   _____   _____
   _____   _____

3. List the organization's top three goals.
   1. _____
   2. _____
   3. _____

4. List three marketing objectives that address the organization's top goals.
   1. _____
   2. _____
   3. _____

5. Choose one marketing objective.

   _____

6. Define the target market(s).

   _____
   _____

7. Determine target market wants and needs.

   _____
   _____

8. Market research techniques to investigate the marketing objective:
   –Demographic analysis   –Consumer preference analysis
   –Focus groups   –Computer analysis
   –Surveys—mail   –Man-on-the street interviews
   –Surveys—telephone   –Personal interviews

9. Competitor analysis:
   Strengths   *Weaknesses*

   _____   _____
   _____   _____
   _____   _____

10. Marketing tactics:
    _____ Logo   _____ Internal marketing
    _____ Image   _____ Personal selling
    _____ Brochure   _____ Advertising
    _____ Newsletter   _____ Direct mail
    _____ Media interviews
    _____ Telecommunications

continues

Exhibit 2-8 continued

---

11. Create a flowchart for the marketing tactics.

12. Market research techniques to evaluate plan effectiveness:
    –Demographic analysis   –Consumer preference analysis
    –Focus groups   –Computer analysis
    –Surveys—mail   –Man-on-the street interviews
    –Surveys—telephone   –Personal interviews

---

2. Describe the external business environment, the market research that was conducted should make it possible to list the opportunities and constraints that exist in a business environment locally and nationally. Factors that affect the external business environment include economic trends, technological trends, consumer attitudes and opinions, and government regulations.
3. List three of the organization's major goals. They should be included in the market plan to ensure that the marketing activities performed throughout the year are actually directed and focused at these goals.
4. List three marketing objectives that address the organization's top goals. Marketing objectives differ from organizational goals in that they are more specific and oriented toward the marketplace.
5. Select one marketing objective from the three listed previously. (Eventually, steps 6 through 12 of the market plan will be completed for each of the marketing objectives listed in step 4.)
6. Define the market's most appropriate target.
7. Determine what that market wants and needs from the clinic or service. Initially, do this by intuitively attempting to elicit the target market's perceptions. Once hunches and guesses have been made about the target market, verify them through market research.
8. Use market research techniques to investigate the marketing objectives. List the market research techniques that can be used for these investigations of the market plan.
9. Perform a competitor analysis in order to determine the strengths and weaknesses of each competitor so that the organization can determine its own differential advantage in the marketplace.

Once these nine steps have been completed, management is finally ready to establish the marketing mix, the tactics to be used in order to accomplish the marketing goals. The marketing mix combines marketing tactics from public relations, advertising and selling, and internal marketing to meet the marketing goals strategically.

10. List the tactics that can be used to accomplish the marketing objective based on the information presented in the market plan. Note the personnel

who will be responsible for these marketing tactics, the budget that will be necessary, and the time frame within which these tasks are to be accomplished.

11. Create a flowchart for these marketing tactics, taking into consideration both ongoing and new marketing activities. Involve all staff members who will be performing marketing activities in steps 10 and 11 in order to increase their enthusiasm and cooperation in the program.

12. List the market research techniques that can be used to evaluate the market plan's effectiveness. Simply accomplishing marketing activities in and of itself does not guarantee success—success is measured through market research techniques.

Exhibit 2-9 is an example of a completed market plan for an outpatient physical therapy clinic that wanted to increase total patient volume and, thus, profitability by offering women antepartum and postpartum services. The clinic had extra space and sufficient staff to treat these patients, although the staff required additional training through reading and attendance at seminars on obstetrics and gynecology. The obstetrician-gynecologists in the community considered low back and wrist pain during pregnancy self-limiting and, therefore, did not commonly refer their pregnant patients to physical therapy. Many professional women in the community wanted to work as long into their pregnancy as possible, were not willing to quit work early because of back pain, and were sometimes being referred for physical therapy through their internists. No one in the community had yet instituted a similar program, but a nearby hospital was considering it.

Exhibit 2-9 Market Plan for Physical Therapy Clinic Preparing To Offer Antepartum and Postpartum Services

---

1. Describe the internal business environment.

Strengths	*Weaknesses*
Sufficient space and equipment	Staff needs specific seminars on the topic
Enthusiastic well-trained staff	topic
Good teamwork between employees	Inexperience marketing to OB-GYN physicians

2. Describe the external business environment.

Opportunities	*Threats*
Women need and want the service	Women don't know of service existence
Internists will refer	Nearby hospital may open similar program
Increased assertiveness of professional women	program
	OB-GYN physicians don't perceive a problem

continues

Exhibit 2-9 continued

3. List the organization's top three goals.

   1. Increase profitability
   2. Increase patient volume
   3. Increase visibility in community

4. List three marketing objectives that address the organization's top goals.

   1. Learn all about the potential market
   2. Institute awareness compaign
   3. Bring target market to a decision to use the service

5. Choose one marketing objective.

   Bring target market to a decision to use the service

6. Define the target market(s).

   OB-GYN physicians

7. Determine target market wants and needs.

   Deliver healthy babies
   Ensure satisfied customers

8. Market research techniques to investigate the marketing objective:

   _Demographic analysis   _Consumer preference analysis
   _Focus groups   _Computer analysis
   √Surveys—mail   _Man-on-the-street interviews
   √Surveys—telephone   √Personal interviews

9. Competitor analysis:

Strengths	*Weaknesses*
Large market budget	Bureaucracy slows decision making
High visibility in community	Less personalized service
Easy access to OB-GYN physicians	No space for the program

10. Marketing tactics:

   _Logo   √Internal marketing
   √Image   √Personal selling
   _Brochure   _Advertising
   _Newsletter   √Direct mail
   _Media interviews
   √Telecommunications

Exhibit 2-9 continued

11. Create a flowchart for the marketing tactics.

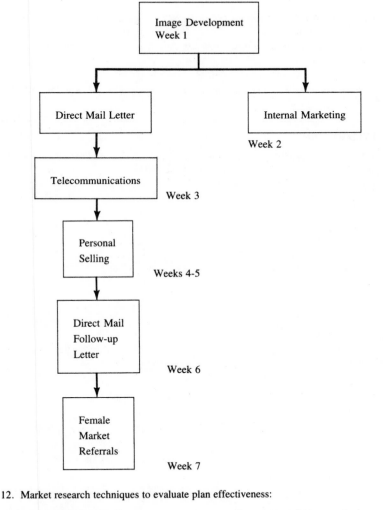

12. Market research techniques to evaluate plan effectiveness:

_Demographic analysis   _Consumer preference analysis
_Focus groups   _Computer analysis
√Surveys—mail   _Man-on-the-street interviews
√Surveys—telephone   √Personal interviews

NOTES

1. *Webster's Ninth New Collegiate Dictionary* (Springfield, Mass.: Merriam-Webster, Inc., 1984), 898.

2. B.E. Johnston and P.J. Lord, *Your Private Practice "Planning and Organization"* (Lake City, FL: Peter J. Lord and Associates, 1982), 4.

3. P. Kotler and R.N. Clarke, *Marketing for Health Care Organizations* (Englewood Cliffs, N.J.: Prentice-Hall, Inc., 1987).

4. Ibid.

5. L. Henderson, *All about Focus Groups: A User's Perspective* (Chevy Chase, Md.: RIVA, Inc., 1989).

SUGGESTED READING

Cooper, PD, Jones, KM, and Wong, JK. *An Annotated and Extended Bibliography of Health Care Marketing*. Chicago: American Marketing Association, 1984.

chapter 3

Internal Marketing: Marketing from the Inside-Out

"You never get a second chance to make a first impression."
1989 Television Ad

The person who waited for a special occasion to entertain at a prestigious restaurant that advertises "luxury dining in elegant surroundings" only to find that the head chef was out sick that day and a convention of shoe salesmen had taken over the main dining room is unlikely to return to that restaurant. Furthermore, that person is likely to tell twenty people of this disappointing experience. (The person who had a good experience is likely to tell only five people.) This poor experience, if substantiated by the experiences of others over time, will create the restaurant's image in the community. No amount of expensive marketing or advertising can overcome a poor product or service.

Customer experience can make or break external marketing efforts. The management of the business functions that, combined, create the customer's experience is called internal marketing. This process ensures that all aspects of the product or service provided match the claims made in external promotions. Congruence between external and internal promotions is the foundation of long-term success.

The goal of all marketing efforts by a physical therapy clinic is to bring those in the target market through the hierarchy of effects until they reach the point of repeat use and recommendation of the clinic. It is easier, less costly, and requires significantly less time to promote word-of-mouth sales to current consumers than it is to promote the service to a completely new market source. Current users of the service are familiar with and understand certain aspects of physical therapy already and, therefore, require less marketing effort to maintain and encourage their satisfaction and repeat use. Any time or money spent on advertising, public relations, and sales efforts is completely wasted, however, unless the clinic provides high-quality therapy. Without such high-quality services, there will be no positive word of mouth, and the clinic will have to rely continually on marketing efforts to bring in new patients just to maintain its existence, not to mention become larger and more profitable.

CUSTOMER SATISFACTION

A satisfied patient population is the foundation of a successful clinic. Word-of-mouth promotions can be the most powerful marketing tool of all.[1] Recommendation by a friend, neighbor, or relative, for example, is still the primary way that consumers choose physicians.[2] Internal marketing is the organization's way of influencing word-of-mouth promotions. Over time, word of the satisfaction level of the clinic's patients spreads to all the target markets, including referring physicians, insurance companies, employers, and even, occasionally, the government. Constant measurement of patient satisfaction should, therefore, be a cornerstone of all marketing efforts.

One technique to determine patient satisfaction is to survey all patients at the time of their discharge from therapy (see Exhibit 3-1). Another technique is to perform a point-in-time interview study, requesting brief answers to questions put to patients who have recently attended therapy; this is sometimes done in a focus group. Still another technique is to place a suggestion comment box near the reception desk with paper, pen, and a sign requesting comments. Both positive and negative comments should be invited. Post positive comments as a staff reward. Follow-up negative comments with actions to correct and change underlying problems. Patients should be informed of these changes to show that staff members care about patients' concerns. The comments and changes should be reviewed on a monthly schedule to help managers keep their fingers on the pulse of the clinic as comments change or stay the same.

It is helpful in designing an internal marketing strategy to know the characteristics of a health care service that contribute to patient satisfaction (Exhibit 3-2). In general, patients respond positively to understandable medical explanations, quality time and quality techniques, as well as a pleasant and empathic personality. Patients also respond positively to a friendly and caring attitude from the ancillary staff, including the receptionist and the aides. Competence in billing and scheduling procedures, responsiveness to needs, an ability to communicate well, and follow-up with requests are needed.[3]

Patient satisfaction is based primarily on subjective feelings of personal interactions and communications rather than a true evaluation of knowledge and skills. Patients do not have the tools for an objective assessment of a professional's credentials, background, and schooling. Therefore, they rely on actions that evoke trust, loyalty, and understanding. Although satisfaction depends primarily on

Exhibit 3-1 Patient Survey

Date _____

Name _____

Dear Patient:

Thank you for choosing our clinic. Your comments about the clinic are important to us. To assist us in our efforts to improve our services, please take a few minutes to answer the following questions. Thank you for your assistance.

1. Was this your first visit to our clinic? _____ yes _____ no
2. Were you aware of our clinic before your physician referred you here?
   _____ yes _____ no
   If yes, how did you hear of us? _____
3. Was this your first experience with physical therapy?
   _____ yes _____ no
4. Which features of our clinic influenced you to use our services?
   Please rate the following in importance to you.

	Very Important	Somewhat Important	Not Important
a) Location	_____	_____	_____
b) Cost	_____	_____	_____
c) All professional staff	_____	_____	_____
d) Doctor expressed preference	_____	_____	_____
e) Reputation in community	_____	_____	_____
f) Hours of service	_____	_____	_____

5. How long on the average did you have to wait in the reception area?
   Less than 5 min., _____ 5–15 min., _____ 15–30 min., _____ 30 + min. _____
6. From your experience in our clinic, please rate the following:

	Excellent	Good	Average	Poor
a) Reception	_____	_____	_____	_____
b) Parking facilities	_____	_____	_____	_____
c) Waiting area	_____	_____	_____	_____
d) Payment procedures	_____	_____	_____	_____
e) Cost	_____	_____	_____	_____

7. How well did the care you received meet your expectations?

   Exceeded expectations _____ Met my expectations _____
   Did not meet my expectations at all _____
   If you found any services lacking, what would you like to see included? _____

8. Did the receptionist:
   a) Greet you pleasantly _____ yes _____ no
   b) Handle payment efficiently _____ yes _____ no

Exhibit 3-1 continued

---

  c) Seem to be (check all that apply)

     Competent _____   Concerned _____   Disrespectful _____

     Courteous _____   Inefficient _____   Unconcerned _____

     Other _____

9. Did the therapist:

  a) Introduce him/herself _____ yes   _____ no

  b) Seem to be (check all that apply)

     Knowledgeable _____   Concerned _____   Incompetent _____

     Aloof _____   Abrupt _____   Informative _____   Courteous _____

     Other _____

10. On a scale of 1–5, how would you rate the overall services of this clinic?

5	4	3	2	1
Excellent	Above Average	Average	Below Average	Poor

11. Would you return to our clinic in the future? _____ yes   _____ no

12. Would you recommend us to a friend or relative?

  _____ yes   _____ maybe   _____ no

13. Comments: _____

_____

_____

Thank you for responding to this questionnaire. Please feel free to call us if you have any other comments you wish to discuss.

---

outcome, patients understand that even the best medical care may not always result in complete wellness. Patients want to understand in their own terms why they are not well, what caused the sickness, and how they can improve and/or live with the condition, however. Their degree of satisfaction drops significantly when these questions are left unanswered.

It is equally important to be aware of factors that lead to patient dissatisfaction. A survey performed of patients in hospitals found that their three leading complaints about their care were:

- the failure of physicians to provide complete explanations
- the lack of consideration from staff members
- requests for personal information within the hearing of others.[4]

Making intangible service benefits appear more concrete and apparent can significantly improve patient satisfaction. For example, it is difficult for patients to recognize advanced professional training unless it is emphasized in a tangible way. Diplomas, licenses, and advanced training certificates can be displayed on the wall. Copies of articles written by staff members and published in professional journals can be placed in the reception area. The benefits of advanced training can

Exhibit 3-2 Patient Satisfying Characteristics

Health Care Provider	Staff
• Comprehensible Explanations	• Friendly Attitude
• Quality Time	• Caring Attitude
• Quality Technique	• Competence
• Pleasant Personality	• Responsiveness
• Empathic Personality	• Good Communication Skills

be highlighted in brochures and newsletters, thus bringing a nontangible service feature to patients' attention in a way that makes it tangible. If advanced training of staff members is an advantage of the clinic over competing clinics, which may hire primarily new graduates, the challenge is to make this advantage obvious and understandable to patients.

IMAGE

Physical therapists should project an image of caring and quality service. These features are extremely intangible, however, and different people perceive and quantify them very differently. Nevertheless, patients will draw conclusions about the quality and level of caring expressed in a clinic. These conclusions will result from tangible measures, such as how much personalized attention they received from the physical therapist, how clean the facility was, how long they had to wait, whether they were greeted with a smile, if their bill was explained with tact, and how pleasant all personnel were. Attention to small details conveys a sense of personal pride and professionalism that makes the therapists' image alive and tangible.

Recognizing the image that the clinic projects is one of the first steps of internal marketing. Because staff members become familiar with their own environment, they often have a biased perspective about its image. It is essential to observe the clinic from an objective point of view, however. The image projected by the clinic springs from a composite of factors, including telephone manners, office cleanliness, billing procedures, and professional treatment.

Visual Impression

Whether the staff is aware of it or not, a clinic's image is always assessed by its target markets. Image is simply a visual impression that cues a person to other responses. "An image is the sum of beliefs, ideas and impressions that a person has of an object."[5] If it were not for their ability to use images to draw conclusions every day, people would be overwhelmed or even threatened by the tremendous confusion and clutter in their minds. Imagine how dangerous it would be if a person who was walking down a city street did not quickly recognize as a threat the image of a powerfully built young man who had an angry expression on his face and was carrying a knife in his hand!

Advertisers know that different segments of the population identify with different images. The agency that manages the advertising for Marlboro cigarettes, for example, recognizes that certain cigarette smokers perceive themselves with a male, macho image. Therefore, it advertises these cigarettes by showing a macho, virile man on horseback riding through the countryside. The subconscious message transmitted through that image appeals to some cigarette smokers.

The challenge of internal marketing is to design a clinic image that positively reflects the service. Therapists assess the image that their patients present as they walk into the clinic, as they smile or frown, and as they sit down. Before patients even say a word, the therapist has begun to draw some conclusions about them, their disability, their emotions, and their reactions. It is naive to believe that the opposite does not also happen. Patients draw conclusions about therapists as professionals and particularly about the quality of care that they will receive at the therapists' hands even before a word is spoken.

Patients begin to draw these conclusions during their initial conversation with the receptionist to make an appointment. This image further develops as they enter the clinic. Impressions are drawn from a combination of the clinic's location in the community, accessibility by public or private transportation, parking facilities, and the building itself, including its lighting and even the smell. These images are confirmed or reassessed as they enter the office and are greeted by the receptionist. The amount of time that they have to wait and the other people who are waiting with them also create an impression of the quality of the service that they may receive. By the time that they watch the therapist walk toward them, greet them, and take them into a treatment room, they have already developed a firm image of the level of professionalism and the quality of service at the clinic. Of course, patients are no more consciously aware that they are drawing these conclusions than people are consciously aware of the conclusions that they make all day based on the images around them.

Definition of Physical Therapy

Studies that a public relations firm has done for the Private Practice Section of the American Physical Therapy Association (APTA) have demonstrated that the public does not have a preexisting image of physical therapists. All therapists have had experiences that indicate this to be true. Students who tell people that they are going into the field of physical therapy usually receive an inaccurate response. When I tell people that I am a physical therapist, the common reaction is, "Oh, I could use a massage." or "Oh, what is a physical therapist?" People are often surprised when I tell them that I treat athletic injuries. All of these comments reflect an incomplete understanding of what physical therapy is.

It is difficult to describe in a few words the breadth and scope of physical therapy as a profession. Physical therapists provide health care services to a broad range of populations with a broad range of disabilities. Therapists are hands-on, high-touch professionals who provide highly individualized and personalized services in pediatrics, sports medicine, oncology, geriatrics, cardiology, orthopedics, obstetrics/gynecology, and neurology. The public cannot really be expected to know anything about physical therapy, because physical therapists have not been very vocal about their profession in the past. It is time for therapists to become vocal. In order to do this, they must be able to describe physical therapy in a few sentences.

The clinic staff can determine what physical therapy means to them and how they can best describe their clinic's service by completing the written exercise in Exhibit 3-3. Although a single therapist can do this exercise, it is preferable to

---

Exhibit 3-3 Image Exercise

Physical Therapy Description

1. List all of the adjectives that describe physical therapy to you.

___	___	___	___
___	___	___	___
___	___	___	___
___	___	___	___
___	___	___	___

2. Select the top ten adjectives that describe physical therapy.

___	___	___	___
___	___	___	___
___	___	___	___

3. Select the top three adjectives that describe your particular clinic.

___	___	___

Exhibit 3-4 Completed Image Exercise

Physical Therapy Description

1. List all of the adjectives that describe physical therapy to you.

professional	caring	motivating	goal-oriented
high-touch	communicative	positive	highly trained
rehabilitative	quality time	progressive	knowledgeable
preventive	friendly	consumer-oriented	long-term value
educational	informative	receptive	healthy

2. Select the top ten adjectives that describe physical therapy.

rehabilitative	high-touch	quality time	motivating
progressive	consumer-oriented	caring	informative
communicative	receptive	highly trained	knowledgeable

3. Select the top three adjectives that describe your particular clinic.

progressive	high-touch	quality time

---

perform it with a group of physical therapists, such as co-workers or classmates. The more physical therapists who are involved, the more creative and effective the outcome will be. Exhibit 3-4 shows a completed exercise.

Once the staff's perceptions of physical therapy have been revealed, the validity of these perceptions can be tested by asking patients what they think. Current patients may be asked to list the first three adjectives that come into their minds when they are asked to describe the clinic (Exhibit 3-5). Predetermining the patients to be asked, without regard to who they are, ensures that the sample is random. For example, every other patient who arrives for treatment, the last patients in the evening, or even the first patients in the morning can be asked. It is important not to bias the sample selection by choosing only patients whom staff members know well.

Once the adjectives that the staff used to describe their perceptions of the physical therapy clinic have been matched with those that patients used to describe their point of view, the results should be compared with the APTA's definition of physical therapy.

> Physical therapy is a health profession whose primary purpose is the promotion of optimal human health and function through the application of scientific principles to prevent, identify, assess, correct, or alleviate acute or prolonged movement dysfunction. Physical therapy encompasses areas of specialized competence and includes the development of new principles and applications to more effectively meet existing and

Exhibit 3-5 Image Development

Ask three patients per day for the next two weeks to list the first three adjectives that come into their minds when you ask them to describe your clinic.

_____   _____   _____

_____   _____   _____

_____   _____   _____

_____   _____   _____

_____   _____   _____

_____   _____   _____

_____   _____   _____

_____   _____   _____

_____   _____   _____

emerging health needs. Other professional activities that serve the purpose of physical therapy are research, education, consultation, and administration.[6]

Image Marketing

In marketing efforts, all three perspectives—the staff's, the patients', and the APTA's—can be used to describe the clinic. Descriptions for different target markets may vary somewhat, because image features may vary in importance to physicians, patients, and insurance carriers. For example, if the clinic's three major image characteristics are (1) advanced skills; (2) high-touch, personalized focus; and (3) cost-effectiveness, newsletters written for the three groups should emphasize different benefits. While advanced skills and training are of primary concern to physician groups, the high-touch, personalized focus is of primary importance to patients. Insurance companies respond best to marketing efforts that emphasize cost-effectiveness. All three benefit features can be discussed in each newsletter, but the emphasis should vary from market to market.

A newsletter targeted to patients could headline a story by a patient about the clinic's personalized service, in which the patient describes how the staff went a step beyond expectations and helped the patient to a faster recovery. A photograph of the patient undergoing treatment or talking to the therapist would bring home the message of the article while promoting the high-touch focus of the clinic. Other articles in the newsletter could emphasize the clinic's cost-effectiveness and the advanced training of the staff. Alternatively, if the newsletter audience is the physician target market, the headline article could feature a new electrical stimulation unit and the advanced seminar attended by a staff therapist. The article could list appropriate referral diagnoses and the expected benefits of the new treatment in order to attract physician interest while highlighting the clinic staff's expertise. The newsletter targeted to insurance claims persons would catch their attention with the headline ''New Billing Procedures Cut Costs at Physical Therapy Clinic.'' This article could be followed by a shorter version of the patient testimonial that focused on the high-touch, personalized service. A shorter version of the benefits of electrical stimulation may also be of interest to this target market. Table 3-1 is an example of image priorities based on differing target market perspectives. Target market priorities can change over time or vary with different specific groups, however, so it is important to research each local target market's priorities.

Newsletters are only one way to use the clinic's top three primary image benefits as the promotional basis of marketing efforts. In combination with an understanding of the wants and needs of the target markets, these benefits make up the cornerstone of all marketing efforts, including brochure development, public speeches, media interviews, sales calls, and even advertising. Therefore, all strategic market planning should begin with an image assessment to establish the three primary benefits to be promoted.

Planning in this fashion ensures clarity of image and honesty in advertising that will be substantiated when patients use the service. It also prevents a common marketing mistake, which is to promote service features that may not be valid. Without research, it cannot be determined whether the clinic actually provides the benefit or even if the target market is actually interested in the benefit. Many clinic brochures that are targeted to everyone, physicians and patients alike, feature benefits that are of more interest to physical therapists than to anyone else. Features such as modalities available, schools attended, continuing education courses listed, and honors received all fall in this category.[7] Physical therapists may think of these benefit features first, but such features are probably not of primary interest to the target market. The only way to know for sure is to research interests in the target market.

Table 3-1 Image Priorities Based on Target Market Perspectives

Physicians	Patients	Insurance Companies
1. Advanced skills	1. High touch	1. Cost-effectiveness
2. High touch	2. Advanced skills	2. Advanced skills
3. Cost-effectiveness	3. Cost-effectiveness	3. High touch

IMAGE BUILDING

Two factors converge to establish a physical therapist's personal professional image as well as the clinic's image in the mind of consumers. One is the object-determined image; the other is the person-determined image.[8] The first is the image obtained from the objective characteristics of an object. If a clinic is modern, tastefully furnished, and impeccably clean, most people conclude that the clinic has a professional appearance. Different people with varying backgrounds and expectations will draw the same conclusions about an object-determined image. The person-determined image, however, is based on subjective characteristics; different people process the same information differently based on their backgrounds and their personalities. For example, if the same clean and modern clinic was crowded with people in the reception area, one person may consider the clinic professional for its cleanliness, while another may consider it unprofessional for its crowds.

In understanding and developing their own personal and clinic image, physical therapists must recognize that both object-determined and person-determined factors influence images. The goal is to create an image that varies as little as possible from person to person, a primarily object-determined image, by maintaining consistent standards of personal and service performance throughout the organization. Consumer feedback should be monitored through patient satisfaction surveys, informal questioning of random patients, and a receptivity to criticism as an opportunity to improve. An organization's image is made up of the personal image created by the staff and the facility image.

Personal Professional Image

A member of the general public who is asked to describe the personal professional characteristics projected by a lawyer, a physician, a pharmacist, or a teacher can easily come up with a number of image descriptions specific to the profession. That same person may find it more difficult to describe a physical therapist, however. Not only are there fewer physical therapists in the population, but also physical therapy is a relatively new profession, having begun only in the 1920s. A large percentage of patients are encountering a physical therapist for the first time. These patients draw conclusions about their therapist and generalize them to the rest of the physical therapy profession. As a result, each physical therapist has a great responsibility, as well as a tremendous opportunity, to shape public opinion about the profession.

Physical therapists should compare the three primary image characteristics that describe physical therapy to them with their own personal image to determine whether there is a match. Any contradiction between the two images will create confusion in the minds of the market group. For example, patients may find it difficult to follow the advice of a sports physical therapist who is overweight and smokes. They will have a problem trusting the treatment program of a professional who looks sloppy, and they will have trouble taking seriously a professional who dresses as if ready to wash a car.

Salespeople know that a client who meets them for the first time draws conclusions about their professionalism, intelligence, and the value of their product within thirty seconds. Once made, these first impressions are difficult to change. It seems unfair that thirty seconds can have such an impact, as this impression can have very little to do with training, experience, and product usefulness; however, everyone draws conclusions about people in this way, thus reducing information clutter and overload. Once physical therapists understand that their personal professional interactions are also subject to first impressions, they can benefit from sales training to build a first impression image that corresponds to their training and knowledge, as well as the treatment that the patient will ultimately receive.

To assess and build a personal professional image that is congruent with their own assessment of the image of physical therapy, physical therapists can begin with the seven image-building strategies taught to professional salespersons.

1. posture
2. grooming
3. fashion
4. visual communication
5. verbal communication
6. nonverbal communication
7. attitude

Posture

Physical therapists know the importance of posture for structure and function. Faulty posture causes muscle imbalance, movement dysfunction, and, ultimately, pain syndromes. Posture also contributes significantly to one person's first impression of another. Different postures indicate different personality characteristics. Others perceive those who hold themselves in a stiff military posture as having rigid, inflexible personalities and those who sit and stand with rounded shoulders and head bent slightly forward as having low self-esteem and/or as being subject to depression. A posture that is out of balance gives the impression of a personality that may be out of balance. To create a positive professional first impression, physical therapists must make their posture work for them psychologically, as well as physically.

Grooming

Because grooming is a very personal and intimate subject, it may be difficult to discuss guidelines for physical therapists. Hair style, fingernail care, and makeup (for women) are some of the first things noticed about a therapist, however. Grooming styles that are appropriate for therapists vary, depending on the location and the demographics of the patient population. Clean, healthy hair in a modern, but not too trendy, cut is usually advisable. Men and women both need to manicure their nails to make sure that they are clean and not too long; moreover, ragged or uneven fingernails on a touching professional indicate a lack of attention to detail and caring. Physical therapists should reflect on the desirable image characteristics of those in their profession and should try to match their look to those characteristics.

Fashion

In a very subtle way, fashion and dress distinguish an individual's self-image and type of work. On the job, many therapists wear a white laboratory coat or jacket. Patients are accustomed to white as the medical professional's dress, and, thus, white inspires trust. Surveys of patients over sixty-five years of age have found that this demographic group generally expect medical personnel to wear white; they have great difficulty trusting a medical professional who does not wear a white laboratory coat or uniform. On the other hand, children are often afraid of white uniforms and respond better to physical therapists who wear street clothes. A survey of teaching hospitals in Boston and San Francisco revealed patients preferences include more formal attire and etiquette than are currently the norm. Development of high standards, they believe, "have considerable impact on effectiveness as physicians, because the verbal and non-verbal interactions between physicians and patients may strongly influence patient compliance and satisfaction."[9] It showed that sixty-five percent felt that physicians seeing a patient should wear white coats. A mere seven percent disagreed with the idea that physicians should wear one during a patient visit. However, twenty-three percent of the physicians surveyed stated that they never wore one, and seventy-two percent of the staff physicians do not always wear one when seeing patients. Less than half of those surveyed felt sneakers were acceptable for a physician to wear when seeing a patient, but forty-three percent of them reported doing so. Fifty-three percent felt blue jeans were not acceptable for a physician seeing a patient. Nine percent of responding physicians wore blue jeans at least some times.[10]

Physical therapists should dress carefully, based on the purpose of their activities. Most male physical therapists are appropriately dressed with a laboratory jacket, shirt and tie, solid color pants, and dark shoes. The therapist who works primarily with an athletic team may be more comfortable working in a sport shirt, however. A change of clothes to a well-tailored suit and tie would be advisable for lunch with a banker or supervising administrator.

When dressing for a meeting with a referral source, a therapist should try to match the style of dress that the referral source is likely to be wearing. A rule of thumb is not to dress more formally or expensively than the person who may bring business to the clinic. Two consultants from New York City dressed in their best three-piece suits when they flew in a private jet to work for a Texas banker noted as their plane landed that the banker was dressed in jeans and a leather vest. They quickly removed their vests and ties and, as they were the same size, switched jackets to look more casual and comfortable for their interaction.

The selection of appropriate dress for female physical therapists is more complicated because of the greater variability of women's styles. Many female physical therapists are turning to wardrobe consultants to help them design the most cost-effective wardrobe for their life style and business needs. A therapist can accessorize a comfortable, well-made pants suit that is suitable for patient care with belt, earrings, and jacket for lunch with a referral source or change the pants to a skirt for an after work professional meeting.

During working hours, the dress of a physical therapist who provides pediatric services usually differs from the dress of a therapist who performs industrial ergonomic assessments. The needs of the client, as well as the focus of the clinic, dictate such differences to a great extent. Running shoes and a warm-up suit may be appropriate for some sports clinics during patient treatment, but, to the general public and to most referral sources, this attire projects a carefree, leisure-time attitude.

Like grooming, fashion makes a statement about a therapist and creates an image. Therapists must be conscious of the fashion statement that they make to their patients, supervisors, and contacts in the community. Building trust is a critical factor in the image that patients hold of a therapist's professional abilities. Trust does not, however, "appear in a patient's heart by chance. By choosing what you tell them with your dress, grooming and etiquette, you choose what they believe about you."[11]

Communication

Therapists' visual, verbal, and nonverbal communication styles play a significant role in the image they project. Physical therapists have an advantage in this area over nontrained salespeople, because their daily patient interactions teach them that steady eye contact improves trust. Visual perceptions, as compared to perceptions received from other senses, account for 55 percent of what patients believe about therapists.

> Additionally, eighty-five percent of what we know has come to us through our eyes. We learn more from what we see than what we hear or

touch. Now, as competitive care is converging upon us in full force, we must maximize . . . the unspoken statement and send "messages" consistent with our skills. If we don't, it is more likely that your patients will believe the visual, when visual and verbal conflict.[12]

A therapist's verbal communication skills are honed daily in educating patients about their dysfunction, the care that they need, and the prevention of future problems. The skills that a therapist requires to motivate patients to perform necessary home exercise routines are not unlike the motivational skills that salespeople require. Clear, concise, and confident verbal communication projects a positive professional image. Several organizations have been formed for the purpose of improving verbal communication skills. One of these organizations, the Toastmasters' Club, provides opportunities for practicing prepared and impromptu speaking. The encouragement and criticism given by members of such organizations helps individuals to fine-tune their ability to put thoughts together concisely, persuasively, and/or humorously.

Nonverbal communication also subtly influences the impression that a therapist makes. Patients note whether a therapist is on time for appointments or appears rushed. Patients perceive the time spent with them by physicians who sit down and are not interrupted as longer than the time spent with them by physicians who stand up with one hand on the doorknob and are interrupted—even though the time spent by the former may actually be less. Nonverbal communications play a critical role in consumer decision making.

Because decisions are based on emotions supported by logic, rather than logic itself, the thoughts others have about us are important. Trust, comfort, fear, suspicion are all players in the process of choosing. Decisions to opt for or decline competitive care from or select another similar provider may very well depend on "feel" about the care that they had received from you, your non-verbal communication.[13]

Attitude

An attitude of "up, relaxed, and yes" helps the salesperson remember several critical attitudes. The initialism URY says "you are why" I am here. Like the good salesperson, the good physical therapist knows that the consumer's point of view is the important one. The up in "up, relaxed and yes" suggests the importance of a happy, friendly manner; a relaxed manner projects self-confidence, and the yes suggests a positive, "can-do" attitude.[14]

Personal Image-Building Strategies

Physical therapists can learn from the image-building strategies taught to salespeople and use them to assess and develop a personal image that is congruent with their image of physical therapy as a profession and of their clinic specifically. The enforcement of these standards on all staff in the clinic can be very beneficial. ''Many major corporations will tell you that, when image standards are adhered to, productivity increases.''[15] Health practitioners who maintain image standards in their practices find ''their patients and peers to have greater respect for them and often having higher expectations, themselves, of their abilities.''[16]

Personal image is an intimate, personal concept. The marketing concept of image building brings therapists out of their perceptions of self and helps them see themselves as others do. Because others' perceptions of therapists are often quite different from therapists' own perceptions, feedback from others' responses to interactions can be very helpful. Colleagues are likely to tell therapists of their strengths selectively, however, tactfully ignore weaknesses. Even so, it is important to get positive feedback about strengths so that they can then be used in marketing efforts. An exercise to determine personal image strengths is to have each person at a staff meeting stand up, turn to the person sitting next to him or her, and list three major personal strengths of that person in terms of image (Exhibit 3-6). With knowledge of their three major image strengths, therapists can promote themselves, their clinic, and their profession.

When ready for a full image assessment, a therapist should go to a professional image builder. Most major cities have them. Good image building consultants can be found in the Yellow Pages or through the reporters on the local television station.

The professional image that physical therapists personally project is essential to complement their marketing program. Physical therapists' services and selves are the product that they are trying to sell. Therefore, building a personal image is the first step in marketing efforts; the image defines the services to be provided. The positive image adjectives of physical therapy and therapists can be used in different settings, such as work, sales calls, marketing literature, and speeches to clubs, associations, and church groups.

The outcome of these personal promotional efforts for physical therapists is to be constantly aware of their image, to project a positive image, and to be enthusiastic in educating people about the profession. Their personal professional image is the strongest marketing tactic in stimulating repeat use, patient satisfaction, and word-of-mouth promotions.

Exhibit 3-6 Image Development

List three major personal strengths of the person sitting next to you in terms of his or her image.
1. _____ 2. _____ 3. _____

Facility Image

A health care organization's image evolves over time from all interactions between the organization and its publics or target markets. This is in addition to public relations and advertising efforts. "An image is the sum of beliefs, ideas, and impressions that a person has of an object."[17] An internal analysis of the organization's facility from the point of view of the public that it serves and in relation to the organization's mission is the facility aspect of internal marketing; this analysis is one of the ongoing phases of all marketing efforts.[18]

A facility analysis begins with the strategic plan that was previously adopted by the organization. This strategic plan contains the organization's mission statement, goals, and purposes. It is important to keep this mission statement in mind when assessing the facility. For example, if a pediatric facility's mission statement directs the organization to make the facility as comfortable for children as possible, doorknobs and light switches should be placed low to meet the requirement of the mission statement.

Assessing and building facility image as part of a marketing plan is relatively inexpensive, because it involves activities that are performed every day.

Marketing Approach in Everyday Activities

A marketing perspective enhances strategic planning and business management. In fact, it is extremely useful to view several managerial functions as marketing functions:

- facility planning and design
- personnel management
- financial management
- policies and procedures development/enforcement.

A marketing perspective results in a facility designed for the use and convenience of the customer, rather than just the manager and the workers. For example, if market research reveals that physical and verbal privacy during treatment is a primary patient concern, the marketing-oriented manager will design individual patient treatment rooms rather than curtained booths. In this way, the facility itself promotes customer satisfaction.

Taking a marketing approach to personnel management provides a subtle perspective on hiring, training, and managing staff. Because a customer orientation is integral to all staff-client interactions, the manager must screen employee applicants not only for their ability to perform the tasks required competently, but also for their ability to make people feel comfortable, good manners, style of dress, and grooming that conforms to the expectations of the clientele. The manager must also look for an attitude in job applicants that, although sometimes wrong, the customer should always be made to feel right. During employee orientation and training, the manager should encourage and positively reinforce the new employee's willingness to ask customers for satisfaction feedback as an integral part of each task learned. New employee training should also emphasize communication skills, including nonverbal cues, and ways to solicit feedback as a method of informal market research. The marketing-oriented manager asks clients about their satisfaction with staff and incorporates this feedback into performance reviews.

The marketing approach also subtly alters financial management. More dollars are spent up front in market research and demographic analysis in order to prevent costly mistakes in planning. Public relations and advertising consume a significant portion of the budget, with the payback of increased volume. An analysis of customer satisfaction facilitates budget planning by making it possible to direct dollars to areas that make a difference in customer perception of service, clinic image, and overall satisfaction.

Policies and procedures should be developed and enforced based on feedback obtained from all target markets through surveys, one-on-one interviews, and customer statements at the time of service. A handbook of policies and procedures should be developed and reviewed at least annually and during initial training. All policies that pertain to customer relations should be assessed and changed when necessary. For example, if referring physicians consider a clinic's ability to treat patients initially within twenty-four hours of referral important, the clinic will benefit from adopting this policy.

Adopting a marketing approach to management functions brings a shift in managerial focus. Staying close to customer wants and needs, knowing how to satisfy those wants and needs, and managing those wants and needs through routine clinic activities markets a clinic without increases in labor and expense. This shift in managerial focus toward a marketing approach also results in better decisions, because the customer is at the center of all decision making.

Internal Marketing Tips

The daily activities in a clinic constitute the ''product'' to be marketed. Internal activities such as typing reports to physicians, billing insurance companies, and answering the telephone courteously may be more important to the long-term success of a clinic than external marketing efforts. These activities comprise internal marketing, which directly affects word-of-mouth promotions and community reputation. The following six activities can be monitored and tracked in the clinic in order to establish and enhance its internal marketing program:

1. guest relations
2. environment

3. personnel
4. telecommunications
5. policies and procedures
6. letters and forms

Guest Relations. A concept that became popular in hospital customer relations in the late 1970s, guest relations is an approach taken from the hotel business; hotel employees are expected to treat every customer who comes in contact with the hotel as they would treat a guest in their own home. Guest relations is an attitudinal concept that needs to permeate all staff members in their interactions with customers. It requires a helpful attitude toward customers when they call on the telephone, when they come in for their appointments, and when they leave after their physical therapy session. Employee attitudes can be tracked through observation, as well as through the patient satisfaction survey.

Environment. A clinic's environment may enhance the patient's entire experience, detract from the experience, or be neutral. The environment includes smell, furniture, lighting, cleanliness, clutter, location, color scheme, and wall decorations. It is the unseen factor that contributes to the clinic's image, just as cleanliness, hair style, and dress contribute to a therapist's personal image. In designing and establishing a clinic image through the environment, it is helpful to review the image desired, based on the organization's mission statement, and the therapists' personal philosophy of patient care. The environment should portray an image that is congruent with the type of care that patients actually receive in the clinic.

Personnel. In order to ensure that the clinic image and its mission statement are actually conveyed to patients, only people who match the clinic's image should be hired—even when it is difficult to find good employees. Furthermore, managers should treat employees as they want the employees to treat their patients. Initial training is extremely important. A heavy work schedule should not be allowed to get in the way of a comprehensive orientation program, as a good orientation program provides employees with the guidelines that they need to provide services in the desired way. Examples of the expected attitude, interpersonal relations, and professionalism should be included in the program. Anecdotes of the ways in which others have performed are useful.

A procedure manual for the purpose of guiding employees as they begin and continue to work at the clinic should be developed. This manual should be reviewed and evaluated at least annually to ensure that existing office policies are being followed and that any past policies that are no longer pertinent are deleted. It should be used as a reference guide not only to orient new employees, but also to communicate expected standards to current employees when there is question about or deviation from office policies and procedures. A well-written personnel manual avoids confusion and unrealistic expectations concerning how management wishes the staff to behave and interact with customers.

Periodic staff meetings reinforce the initial orientation and encourage a positive team-building spirit congruent with the mission of the organization. Should personal problems arise during a staff meeting, they should be tabled and dealt with privately at a later date. When appropriate, all staff members in attendance at the meeting can be informed of the problem resolution.

Personnel performance in relation to internal marketing needs to be measured through observation, as well as through patient satisfaction surveys.

Telecommunications. The telephone is the clinic's communication link to the outside world, and it can be used to promote and project the clinic's image. Because many people who call may never visit the clinic, they may receive their only impression of the clinic through the telephone call. Therefore, written policies and procedures concerning the appropriate way to answer the telephone and the correct responses to various inquiries are desirable, even in the smallest clinic, to ensure that telephone communications are uniform and consistent. There are several rules of thumb for telephone use.

- Never let the telephone ring more than three times before it is answered.
- Never put someone on hold for more than thirty seconds without returning to assure the caller that he or she has not been forgotten.
- Always assume that the person on the other line is a VIP.

Telecommunications can be tracked in several ways. For example, managers may observe employees within the clinic, or they may make random telephone calls to the clinic from outside to determine if employees are actually following the policies and procedures concerning telephone answering. Another method of evaluating telecommunications is to ask a friend or associate to call as a bogus patient, physician, or insurance claim agent and have that person rate the telephone etiquette based on the clinic's policies and procedures.

Policies and Procedures. In addition to an employee guide and handbook, it is useful to have a policy and procedure manual. A clinic that is located in a hospital, nursing home, or a Medicare-certified, free-standing clinic probably has a policy and procedure manual. This manual contains the written, formal policies and procedures of the activities that occur in the clinic on a routine, day-to-day basis. It should also contain a statement of the clinic's philosophy of patient care and concerns for patient safety.

Every organization also has unwritten policies and procedures. It is management's responsibility to ensure that these unwritten policies and procedures do not veer from the purpose and mission statement of the organization. Individuals who are seeking power and control often shift internal policies and procedures to meet their own personal needs. It is imperative that the manager notes when this happens and takes steps to eliminate this type of behavior, for it will not escape the notice of other staff members and will reduce their ability to function as a team.

Letters and Forms. All letters that are sent from the clinic should conform to a basic format so that the clinic's image is consistent. Letters routinely sent to physicians concerning patient care, as well as form letters to insurance companies concerning claims and to patients concerning billing, should be evaluated, reviewed, and updated periodically by management in order to ensure that they are promoting the desired facility image. In addition, the forms that the patient receives initially, which explain the clinic's services and billing procedures, have an impact on the patient's impression of the clinic. Although it is imperative to clearly state the clinic's financial policies at this time, it is important not to give the impression that finances are the clinic's highest priority. The forms that patients receive on exercise programs should have the clinic's name and telephone number on them; the patients will be (or should be) referring to these forms daily, and it is desirable to keep the clinic name and image in front of them as much as possible.

Letters and forms can be evaluated in several ways. Referring physicians may be asked periodically about the usefulness of the letters that they receive from the physical therapists in the clinic. Additionally, patients in the clinic may be surveyed to determine what they think about the usefulness and the image of the clinic's forms.

Corporate History. Instilling company purpose and vision in employees can be difficult in the best of times, but even more effort must be made in the current employment environment. Employees no longer stay with a company for many years. They may change jobs often to move their careers forward. Furthermore, mergers and acquisitions provide a less than continuous environment for workers. Co-opting employees into the mission and vision that initially made the clinic successful can establish a common thread of purpose among all employees. Capturing corporate history through anecdotes and stories told by the founders can communicate this vision in a colorful and memorable way. "These anecdotes can tell an employee more about company policy than all the memos and procedure manuals put together."[19]

The corporate history can also serve as a marketing tool. Clients remember stories of vision, achievement, and dedication much better than they remember a list of perceived benefits in a traditional marketing package. Brief stories can be included in newsletters, featured on a brochure as a quote, or shared during a sales call or even a chance meeting. Anecdotes can be helpful during proposal presentations to establish rapport with a client and to increase the client's understanding of the reason that the organization was formed. One story is told by a group of physical therapists in private practice who formed a corporation to negotiate contracts with insurance companies. As their first meeting with one of the largest carriers in the area began, the clients acted with formality and reserve. Early in the discussion, one of the presenters explained how the founders met and developed the group. The clients relaxed visibly as they realized that the group's purpose was specifically to negotiate with companies such as theirs.

Corporate anecdotes can be discovered by interviewing the founders about "old times." They may be asked questions such as the following to elicit the corporate history:

- What motivated you to begin this company?
- Do you remember your first marketing efforts? Tell me about them.
- What do you remember about your first clients?
- What mistakes do you wish you hadn't made?
- Tell me about the first staff.

The anecdotes received in response to these questions that best describe the founders' vision and purpose, match the current mission statement, or explain certain policies and procedures can be shared at staff meetings, sprinkled throughout the procedure manual, and incorporated into marketing materials as appropriate.

Self-Assessment

The cost of hiring a marketing consultant to research the facility's image is prohibitive for most physical therapy clinics; however, this is not a reason to avoid facility assessment. Much useful information can be obtained through a self-assessment. Although self-assessment is always biased, involving the clinic's entire staff can help reduce that bias by evoking a wider range of opinion and dialogue.

The purpose of the facility self-assessment is to evaluate the environment from an objective viewpoint. The patient or visitor who is at the clinic only for brief appointments over a finite period of time often has a very different perspective than does the professional who works there. In addition, environmental needs may differ. For example, the patient may need to have the privacy of individual treatment rooms, while the clinic director may need to use curtained booths rather than individual treatment rooms because of space constraints. Professional staff may see the equipment stored in the hallway as part of the furniture, while the patient on crutches may find it difficult to maneuver around the equipment and wonder why it is there. The challenge of a facility self-assessment is for the physical therapists to remove themselves from their own perspective as much as possible.

A facility image incorporates all a client's experiences, including the physical characteristics of the clinic and the attitudes of the staff. To assess a physical therapy clinic, the physical therapists who work there can perform the following exercise individually or, preferably, in a management or staff meeting:

> Take a few minutes to imagine that you are a patient being treated in the clinic for the first time. Close your eyes and imagine yourself calling for an appointment. (*One person reads the questions aloud while the other staff members close their eyes and visualize being a patient.*)

- How is the telephone answered?
- Are you told what to expect concerning your treatment and how long it will take?
- What information are you given about payment?

You are traveling to the facility.

- What means of transportation do you use?
- Is someone bringing you?
- Do you drive yourself?
- Where do you park?
- How do you get from the parking area into the facility?

You arrive at the building.

- Are there automatic doors, or do you have to open them yourself?
- If you open the door, how heavy is it?
- As you walk in, what is your impression of the facility?
- Is it clean—is it new?
- Is it stark?
- Is it welcoming?
- Is it confusing?
- Is it orderly?
- What about the signs?
- Is it clear how to locate your department or clinic?

You arrive at the physical therapy clinic.

- What is your first impression?
- What are the reception procedures?
- Are you supposed to sign in?
- Do you know where to go to sign in?

- How are you greeted?
- Who greets you first?
- Do you have to fill out some forms?
- Do you have to talk about insurance and payment? If so, how is it discussed with you?
- Who brings you to an examination room?
- What does that person tell you to expect?
- Who is the next person you talk to?
- Who tells you to take off your clothes?
- Is your modesty respected when you're taking off your clothes and putting on a gown?
- When you're greeted by the therapist, what does the therapist say?
- What is your impression of the therapist and the clinic?
- Does the therapist seem to have enough time for you?
- How many times is the therapist interrupted during the treatment?
- Are you part of the treatment-planning and goal-setting session?
- Are the results of the evaluation and treatment program thoroughly explained to you?
- Are you asked if you have any questions?
- Are your questions answered?
- When treatment is finished and you're ready to leave, is it clear what to expect after the first visit? More pain, less pain?
- Do you know how to perform the home program that you have been given?
- Do you understand when to come back?
- Do you have to make an appointment?
- Are you comfortable with the way payment was handled?
- Do you feel that you were treated well at your first visit?
- Are you looking forward to coming back?
- Did you enjoy yourself?
- If it wasn't the kind of treatment that you could enjoy, do you at least feel that you were treated as professionally and as appropriately as possible?

Now open your eyes.

Once the visualization aspect of the facility image assessment is completed, each participant should list the positive and negative features that were discovered about the clinic. Then, the individual lists can be combined on a chalkboard or flip chart. As in a brainstorming session, there are no wrong answers. The group then selects the top ten positive features provided; these are the clinic's opportunities, or strong points. The top ten negative features are the clinic's obstacles, or weak points (Exhibit 3-7).

The top three opportunities and obstacles should be selected from the lists of ten on the basis of the factors that consumers find most important in designating quality health care. According to studies performed in 1987, consumers perceive quality in health care as a "concerned and caring attitude."[20] Therefore, the three opportunities selected as quality factors should demonstrate a concerned and caring attitude. These three opportunities are the clinic's consumer benefits. In a determination of the clinic's differential advantage, these consumer benefits are its marketing edge.

Exhibit 3-7 Facility Image Assessment

Opportunities (Positive features of the clinic)	*Obstacles* (Negative features of the clinic)
1. _____	1. _____
2. _____	2. _____
3. _____	3. _____
4. _____	4. _____
5. _____	5. _____
6. _____	6. _____
7. _____	7. _____
8. _____	8. _____
9. _____	9. _____
10. _____	10. _____

Opportunities
Pick the top three opportunities and consider them consumer benefits.

1. _____
2. _____
3. _____

Obstacles
Pick the top three obstacles and develop management strategies to eliminate them.

1. _____
   _____
2. _____
   _____
3. _____
   _____

Similarly, the factors that impede a concerned and caring attitude should be considered the top three obstacles to a positive consumer image of the facility. These are weaknesses that the competition can exploit. Management strategies should be developed to overcome these obstacles.

Exhibit 3-8 is an example of one clinic's completion of the facility image assessment. The clinic staff reviewed the top ten opportunities and obstacles to

Exhibit 3-8 Completed Facility Image Assessment

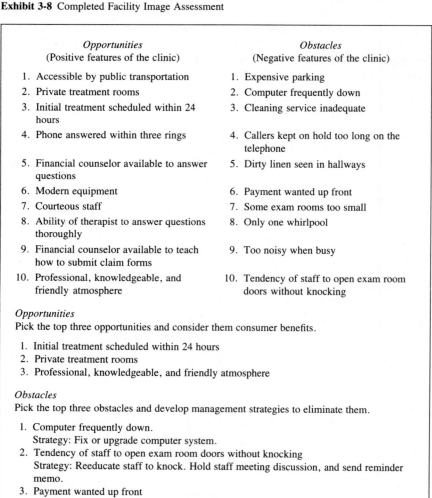

Opportunities (Positive features of the clinic)	*Obstacles* (Negative features of the clinic)
1. Accessible by public transportation	1. Expensive parking
2. Private treatment rooms	2. Computer frequently down
3. Initial treatment scheduled within 24 hours	3. Cleaning service inadequate
4. Phone answered within three rings	4. Callers kept on hold too long on the telephone
5. Financial counselor available to answer questions	5. Dirty linen seen in hallways
6. Modern equipment	6. Payment wanted up front
7. Courteous staff	7. Some exam rooms too small
8. Ability of therapist to answer questions thoroughly	8. Only one whirlpool
9. Financial counselor available to teach how to submit claim forms	9. Too noisy when busy
10. Professional, knowledgeable, and friendly atmosphere	10. Tendency of staff to open exam room doors without knocking

Opportunities
Pick the top three opportunities and consider them consumer benefits.

1. Initial treatment scheduled within 24 hours
2. Private treatment rooms
3. Professional, knowledgeable, and friendly atmosphere

Obstacles
Pick the top three obstacles and develop management strategies to eliminate them.

1. Computer frequently down.
   Strategy: Fix or upgrade computer system.
2. Tendency of staff to open exam room doors without knocking
   Strategy: Reeducate staff to knock. Hold staff meeting discussion, and send reminder memo.
3. Payment wanted up front
   Strategy: Communicate thoroughly, individually, and privately why payment is expected up front and how the patient can submit claims to maximize reimbursement.

select three of each that most significantly affect a consumer's perceptions of a concerned and caring attitude. The three top opportunities were considered this clinic's consumer benefits, and these benefits were highlighted on the clinic's brochure, in its newsletter, in sales calls and speeches, and in all advertising. The three top obstacles were corrected and converted to opportunities through the management strategies developed at the meeting.

Each clinic should go through a process of facility image assessment every six months—more frequently if the clinic is undergoing rapid change. Periodic reassessment is necessary because of the changing nature of every facility's image. The image changes whenever there is a change in any of the facility's variables, such as professional or support staff turnover, increased or decreased patient volume, equipment acquisition or maintenance, insurance reimbursement changes, and staff burnout or enthusiasm. Performing a facility image assessment every six months helps to keep staff and management perceptions of service quality closer to the reality of customer perceptions and expectations. Exhibit 3-9 is a facility image checklist for use with the facility image assessment. Each of these aspects of a facility image should be considered before the facility assessment is completed.

Once the facility self-assessment exercise is completed, the staff as a group can address the following questions to determine clinic attitude:

- What is our appearance? Do we have a uniform? If not, do we have a uniform standard of grooming?
- What level of confidence do we express through nonverbal behavior?
  —facial expressions
  —positive versus negative attitudes
  —enthusiasm
- How do we treat each other in front of the customer?
- What customer interaction habits do we have?
  —a smile
  —listening attentively
  —communicating with our customers

Customer satisfaction surveys can be used to support or refute opinions developed in this way.

Facility self-assessment is the least expensive way to determine facility image. It costs only the time that staff members spend to perform the assessment. The benefits of self-assessment are the verification and clarification of staff perceptions and the sharing of beliefs among staff members. An additional benefit to self-assessment is its use as a personnel management tool. The assessment may help to unify staff members to work toward the same purpose in terms of customer

Exhibit 3-9 Facility Image Assessment Checklist

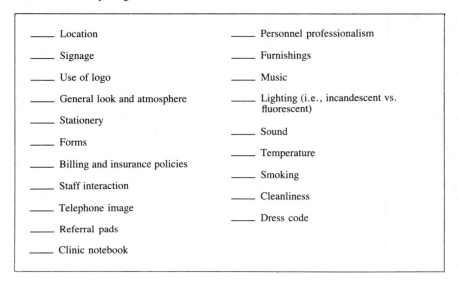

relations. The biggest weakness of self-assessment is the bias held when staff members attempt to assess themselves, as it is difficult for individuals to see their shortcomings objectively.

Use of a Professional Image Consultant

A professional marketing company can perform a complete image assessment at any point in time. The purpose of hiring such a company is to establish a baseline facility image prior to the development of a marketing campaign to change the image so that the subsequent change can be measured. A professional image consultation by a marketing company is expensive, however, and requires a substantial financial commitment to a comprehensive marketing and image-enhancing program. Actual costs can be determined by requesting bids from various firms.

The advantage of a professional image consultation is its objectivity, because it is done by an outside organization without a vested interest in the results. Management should not expect more from a professional image consultation than it is able to provide, however. Knowledge of a facility's image, even changing a facility's image, does not necessarily increase referrals, productivity, or profitability. When managers have false expectations of what a facility image consultation can do for them, the expense of the effort is not justified.

IMAGE MODIFICATION

Although an organization's image is formed and promoted by the owners, managers, and staff, the actual image is held in the minds of consumers. A consumer's image of a health care organization is shaped by many factors, including individual and community beliefs, values, and opinions that vary from person to person and change over time. Those within the organization who manage its image need to stay close to the customers in order to know what their perceptions are and how these perceptions are shifting over time.

If it is discovered that a facility's image is in trouble, the image needs to be modified (Exhibit 3-10). The process of modifying a facility's image involves several steps; it is necessary to

1. describe the desired image characteristic.
2. determine the type of changes that are needed (e.g., staff attitudinal changes or structural changes). It is easier to change attitude problems than facility structural problems.
3. develop strategies for making those changes within the organization.
4. communicate these changes through marketing techniques to the target market.
5. determine the cost.
6. determine the time it will take to change the undesirable image characteristic.[21]

The fact that a facility's image tends to last even if the reality has actually changed can work both ways for a facility. A positive image can linger in people's perceptions long after the quality of care has actually diminished. Eventually, the perceptions will change. Performing the image assessment techniques described in this chapter on a regular basis should help managers recognize when their clinic's image is starting to deteriorate, before it is too late.

Exhibit 3-10 Image Modification

1. Describe the undesirable image characteristic.
2. Describe the desired image characteristic.
3. Determine the type of changes (attitudinal or structural).
4. List the changes that need to be made.
5. List the marketing techniques necessary to communicate these changes to the marketplace.
6. Determine the cost of this image change.
7. Determine the time it will take to make the change and change perceptions in the community.

NOTES

1. S. Brown and A. Morley, *Marketing Strategies for Physicians: A Guide to Practice Growth* (Oradell, N.J.: Medical Economics Company, Inc., 1986), 169–176.

2. D.C. Coddington and K.D. Moore, *Market-Driven Strategies in Health Care* (San Francisco: Jossey-Bass, Inc., 1987), 43–44.

3. S.W. Brown and A.P. Morley, Jr., et al., *Promoting Your Medical Practice* (Oradell, N.J.: Medical Economics Books, 1989), 57, 121.

4. Ibid., 77.

5. Philip Kotler, *Marketing Management*, 5th ed. (Englewood Cliffs, N.J.: Prentice-Hall, Inc., 1984), 68.

6. J. Mathews, ed., *Practice Issues in Physical Therapy* (Thorofare, N.J.: Slack, Inc., 1989), 3.

7. Brown, Morley, et al., *Promoting Your Medical Practice*, 75–87.

8. Philip Kotler and R.N. Clarke, *Marketing for Health Care Organizations* (Englewood Cliffs, N.J.: Prentice-Hall, Inc., 1987), 64.

9. C. Mosbacher, *Images in Health Care* (Washington, D.C.: Aeropolis Books, Ltd., 1987), 121.

10. Ibid.

11. Ibid., 33.

12. Ibid., 27.

13. Ibid., 32.

14. K. Dlemar, *Winning Moves*, (New York: Warner Books, 1984), p 21.

15. Mosbacher, *Images in Health Care*, 19.

16. Ibid.

17. Kotler and Clarke, *Marketing for Health Care Organizations*, 62.

18. R.S. MacStravic, "Professional and Personal Quality of Care in Health Care Delivery," *Health Marketing Quarterly* 5 (1987/88):13, 16.

19. *Marketing News*, December 18, 1989, p 2.

20. Coddington and Moore, *Market-Driven Strategies in Health Care*, 79–80.

21. Kotler and Clarke, *Marketing for Health Care Organizations*, 67.

chapter 4

Public Relations

The public is becoming increasingly hungry for medical information.[1] Since the late 1980s, most evening news programs have included a health spot. Major magazines now carry a regular health feature as well. Newspapers either have a full-time health reporter or feature a health column on a regular basis. Church groups and public service organizations are becoming more interested in health promotion and health information provided through lectures and literature. This increased public interest in medical information gives health professionals an opportunity to publicize their organizations' benefits while providing a community service.

Public relations is the marketing strategy that communicates information about an organization and its purpose or knowledge base in a way that primarily benefits the target market. Secondarily, public relations gains recognition for the organization by promoting its image, name, and primary features. Public relations can be an organization's strategic approach to communication with its target audiences. The message that the organization communicates through public relations is its underlying commitment to professionalism, as well as the benefits and differential advantages of its product. The target audiences are potential patients/clients, physicians, legislators, insurance companies, and businesses identified through the organization's strategic plan. There are various public relations techniques for communication, including, but not limited to, the use of logos, newsletters, brochures, news releases, public speaking, and media interviews.

When used in conjunction with a comprehensive strategic marketing plan, these communication tools can effectively promote an organization. Once the organization's marketing goals, its target markets, the location of the target markets in the hierarchy of effects, and the desired position of the organization among the competition have been identified, an appropriate series of these marketing tools can be selected to reach the organization's marketing goals.

Physical therapists can learn to develop and use the public relations tools by applying techniques that they already know. For example, the use of a brochure in marketing can be analogous to the use of ultrasound in physical therapy. Therapists learn the physical and physiological principles, as well as application techniques, for the use of ultrasound. When this knowledge is combined with a comprehensive evaluation of the patient's condition, the medical diagnoses, and goals for patient outcome, ultrasound is effective and useful. When ultrasound is used on a painful muscle without diagnosis, evaluation, or goal setting, however, it may or may not effectively help the condition. Similarly, therapists must learn how to design, create, and use a brochure by evaluating market conditions, preparing goals, and identifying the desired outcome for the marketing plan if the brochure is to be effective. If a brochure is sent to a potential market without a comprehensive marketing strategy it may or may not result in an effective outcome.

Unlike advertising, which is purchased directly, public relations marketing activities are paid for indirectly.[2] Public relations activities are paid primarily in time, materials, and, sometimes, consultant fees. In general, material produced for public relations is more believable than advertising because it is not produced strictly to sell, but rather to inform. Although the public relations departments of health care organizations have been responsible for communicating opinion, viewpoint, and medical news releases to the media for decades, advertising is relatively new. The introduction of advertising to the health care marketing package in the late 1970s has increased sophistication and proliferation of public relations efforts as comprehensive marketing programs have become the norm for health care organizations.

Public relations efforts will remain a primary marketing strategy and force for health care organizations because of the strength of their impact, targetability, and personal approach. Organizations can design and implement many of their own public relations efforts, which is particularly useful for organizations on tight budgets. The time, materials, and initial mistakes do incur a cost to the organization, however, and should be considered in the budget and annual plan. In this way, it is possible to determine exactly when it is best to hire a consultant, outside public relations firm, or in-house marketing director for assistance in developing logos, newsletters, brochures, or other communication tools.

LOGOS

An organization's logo is a symbolic message designed to elicit instant recognition from the consumer.[3] It should create a unique identity for the organization within today's cluttered informational environment, making the organization stand out from its competitors. In addition, the logo is often the consumer's first impression of a company, organization, or clinic, and first impressions are tremendously important.

Logos are commonly graphic designs or symbols that, over time, come to represent many company attributes or services. For example, the "walking fingers" logo of the Yellow Pages universally represents access to information and help from many businesses. At times, logos may even generate emotions, as the sight of the Easter Seal lily may generate compassion or generosity for disabled children. A strong logo becomes associated with the positive traits and characteristics of the company.

People recognize and are influenced by logos everyday. The image of McDonald's golden arches causes the public to think immediately of fast food, hamburgers, and French fries. McDonald's has effectively positioned those arches in the public mind. In creating a logo for a physical therapy clinic, the goal is the same—to create a symbol that will immediately bring to mind certain images in the person who is exposed to the logo. Images that are associated with physical therapy include strength, movement, or hands.

Benefits of a Logo

There are at least three reasons for a physical therapy clinic to design and use a logo.

1. quick recognition
2. uniqueness
3. graphic identity

A logo should be designed to provide a good first impression that, over time, can be recognized instantly. It helps the target market remember the clinic because it is the clinic's professional image on paper. For quick recognition, it should have a simple, easy-to-remember design and color combination. Because it represents the organization's position in the marketplace and differentiates it from its competitors, the logo design should be unique. Common medical symbols, such as the caduceus or da Vinci's anatomical man, should be avoided, as these symbols are used too frequently to state anything unique and meaningful about an organization. Finally, the logo is the organization's graphic identity and reinforces the benefits that it offers consumers. Therefore, it should be designed to reflect the organization's professional image, the quality features of its product, and the specific attributes of its service. An experienced and creative graphic artist can design a logo that contains these features and will work well for a clinic's image for years to come.

Design of an Effective Logo

A good logo says something true about the clinic as it makes a first impression of the business.[4] The design of the logo symbol and the typeface of the printed message should be consistent and clear. Traditional typeface and stationery should be matched with a traditional symbol. A progressive, innovative symbol should be matched with similar lettering and typeface. Because the choice of color(s) also contributes to the image, it must be made with care.

A good logo should complement the clinic's professional image. An ornate, Old English typeface would not complement a clinic in which the physical therapists are young and progressive. Likewise, a traditional university-based hospital clinic that prides itself on its older, more established physicians and reputation would not benefit from a logo on a nontraditional color of stationery, such as yellow or green.

A good logo should be easy to read and understand. It is the rare person who will look closely enough at a logo to decipher difficult graphics. Printing the clinic slogan or name too small can defeat the purpose. Furthermore, the logo must be simple enough to be used in many sizes. Its message should be clear even when it is reduced small enough to fit on clinic stationery and business cards. It may be reproduced in black and white for a newsletter, telephone book, and newspaper ads. Simplicity that translates into readability and instant recognition is the goal of a logo.

A logo should be printed in the same color each time it is used, unless it is desirable to distinguish different products or service divisions by different colors. Keep in mind, however, that the logo may be reproduced in black and white; therefore, use colors that contrast well. Even in that case, color distinction should be used consistently. If at all possible, logo colors should match the clinic's decor. The image that various colors project must be considered, however. Single colors or color combinations bring forth various images and feelings in the consumer. For example, the mention of a restaurant that uses bright orange and turquoise probably brings Howard Johnson's immediately to mind. Each additional color increases the printing price considerably.

Companies that wish to affiliate their image with traditional U.S. qualities often use the colors red, white, and blue. Health care logos have traditionally avoided red because of its possible association with blood. For this reason, a clinic may still want to avoid a red logo, especially if burn or wound care is one of its specialties. On the other hand, if the clinic is a free-standing outpatient facility that specializes in sports medicine for Olympic athletes, red, white, and blue may be appropriate logo colors. Traditional health care colors are blue and ivory. A physical therapy clinic may want to use or avoid these colors, depending on the traditional or progressive nature of its business. Gold and silver embossing or foil give a logo an exclusive, expensive look, but they do not photocopy well and may not project an appropriate image unless the clinic is an upscale provider. Dark brown or black lettering on a light tan background can look formal and businesslike. If a clinic's image is modern, bold, and cheerful, a white background with primary colored lettering may be the best choice.

Evaluation of Competitors' Logos

Before designing a logo, it is important to learn from the examples of others! Samples of health care and commercial logos should be collected and their impact examined in terms of immediate impressions and feelings. Logos that present an image similar to that of the clinic, as well as logos that present the opposite impression, should be examined. If the clinic's image is contemporary, warm, and progressive, for example, the collection should contain logos that express those qualities, as well as logos that represent a traditional, technical, and conservative image. This collection of logos can be used to distill and develop ideas for the clinic's logo and to share with the graphic designer at the appropriate time. The three steps required to evaluate competing logos are shown in Exhibit 4-1.

Preparation for Logo Design

In starting a new program or opening a new clinic, it is advisable to defer the final design of a logo symbol to represent the product or service. New programs usually undergo tremendous changes during the first six to twelve months of their

Exhibit 4-1 Competitor Logo Evaluation

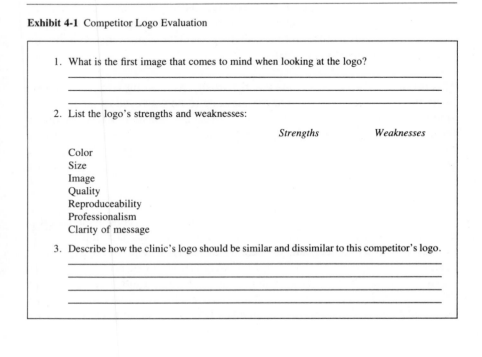

1. What is the first image that comes to mind when looking at the logo?

2. List the logo's strengths and weaknesses:

	Strengths	Weaknesses
Color		
Size		
Image		
Quality		
Reproduceability		
Professionalism		
Clarity of message		

3. Describe how the clinic's logo should be similar and dissimilar to this competitor's logo.

existence, and it may be necessary to alter the symbol originally planned after a year as the program develops into something slightly or perhaps even dramatically different. While waiting to design a logo, management can decide on colors for stationery, a color scheme for the office, and a typeface for the letterhead. The latter can serve as the logo until it is possible to determine the best way to identify the product to the consumer. After the clinic's image and position in the marketplace have been well developed, they will rarely change. At this point, an effective and long-lasting logo can be designed.

If a graphic artist is to design the logo, the clinic representative must be well prepared for the first meeting. A simple four-step preparation process will produce the best results.

1. Send the artist the following documents prior to the first visit:
   a. mission statement
   b. list of image adjectives that describe the clinic
   c. position statement
   d. any brochures or newsletters
   e. definition of physical therapy
2. Collect copies of at least fifty logos. Include the competition's logo, logos from other health care organizations, and contemporary logos from business and industry.
3. Meet with the staff and list the positive and negative aspects of the fifty logos. Relate the comments to the image that the clinic wishes to project.
4. Ask each staff member for ideas that represent the clinic's image. Select the best ideas to show the artist.

This process will reduce the time that the artist/consultant must spend getting to know the clinic, its services, and the message to be conveyed to the audience. Additionally, the more information that the artist has, the more likely that one of the first three designs will be the right logo for the clinic. This is important because the contract usually calls for three choices. Additional logo options are additional costs.

Use of Consultants

Once all of the brainstorming is done, it is time to contact a consultant, usually a graphic artist, to pull the ideas together in a polished way (Exhibit 4-2). The graphic artist should understand the health care field and demonstrate expertise in designing for health care organizations. Otherwise, it may be necessary to spend valuable time to educate the consultant about the field of health care services and the differences from products or other services, and the consultant's designs may be unsatisfactory. It is best to find an artist who has either graphic or personal

Exhibit 4-2 Graphic Consultant Selection

1. Investigate the following resources:
   - Yellow Pages (commercial or graphic artist)
   - advertising agencies specializing in health care
   - large printers
   - universities with schools of graphic design
   - recommendations
2. Conduct an interview to accomplish the following:
   - look for empathy with the mission
   - review portfolio
   - call for references
3. Sign a contract specifying:
   - cost
   - deadlines
   - number of designs
   - who will do the work
4. Work with the graphic consultant to:
   - review the documents sent in the preparation step in person and get the consultant's feedback or understanding of the clinic's service
   - keep in close contact with progress and request preliminary sketches
5. Use the logo consistently and display it prominently on stationery, business cards, signage, and promotional giveaways.

experience with rehabilitation. Samples of the artist's work should be examined to ensure that the style and professionalism are in line with the clinic's needs.

A logical place to start looking for a graphic artist is in the Yellow Pages under commercial artists. Local advertising agencies that specialize in health care advertising may be helpful, but an advertising agency is more expensive than an independent graphic artist and may want to take over some of the background and creative work that has already been done. Often, large printers have in-house graphic artists who could provide a logo. If not, they usually know one or two graphic artists whom they could recommend. Finally, the talent in the design departments of local universities should not be overlooked. Oftentimes, excellent, creative pieces may be obtained for a reduced price from a student.

In the initial discussions, the clinic representative must be sure that the graphic artist understands physical therapy and can empathize with the staff about the services that they are offering in creating a logo. The representative should examine the artist's portfolio carefully and discuss ways in which his or her health care experience and graphics coincide with the clinic's needs. The consultant should be able to recommend the typeface that will most readily convey the kind of message that promotes the clinic most effectively; provide guidance on colors and paper weight; and give assistance in the use of the logo on stationery letterhead, as well as business cards, brochures, and newsletters.

A contract should be finalized only if it specifies costs, deadlines, and the number of designs to be submitted. It should include a clause stating that the person interviewed will do the work. As for any person being hired, references for recommendations from previous jobs should be requested.

Although ''you get what you pay for,'' it is not always the case in this field. The television network NBC, for example, paid more than $500,000 to change its logo to the current design. Simultaneously, a graphics studio designed the exact logo for a small firm in Minneapolis with the initials NBC for a mere $200. In addition to the indirect costs of approximately twenty hours preparation time, a clinic should expect a direct cost between $350 to $2,000 on the consultant's development of its logo. Although there is really no price ceiling on the cost of a logo, a first-rate symbol should be obtained for less than $2,000.

Marketing Uses of the Logo

To be effective as a marketing tool, a logo must be prominently and frequently displayed. It should be incorporated in all marketing efforts; it should be included on all stationery, business cards, signage, and promotional giveaways. If possible, the colors of the logo should be repeated in the office decor for consistency and subconscious identification and recognition. A well-designed logo marketed consistently will come to represent the organization's image, differential advantage, and attributes.

Logo of the American Physical Therapy Association

The American Physical Therapy Association (APTA) restricts the use of its logo. The APTA's policy as promulgated by the Board of Directors in 1982 is as follows:

Policy on Use of the Association's Insignia (Logo),
Name and Address

The Association's insignia (logo) is a registered trademark and the property of the American Physical Therapy Association. The insignia can be used only as designated and approved by the Association. The Association's components may imprint or affix the Association's insignia on or to stationery, publications, documents, and other materials produced by the components, provided that:

1. any such use of the insignia is approved by the component's governing body and by the Executive Director of the American Physical Therapy Association, and
2. the insignia is imprinted or affixed adjacent both to the component's name and to statement of the component's relationship to the Association (e.g., "A Chapter of the American Physical Therapy Association," or "A Section of the American Physical Therapy Association"), and
3. a copy or sample of any such material produced by the component for public relations or public information directed to other than members of the component is sent to the Association's Public Relations Department for informational purposes.

The Association's components may also imprint or affix the Association's full name on or to stationery, publications, documents, and other materials produced by the components, provided that:

1. any such use of the Association's name is approved by the component's governing body, and
2. the Association's name is imprinted or affixed adjacent to the component's name as part of a statement of the component's relationship to the Association (see examples above), and
3. a copy or sample of any such material produced by the component for public relations or public information directed to other than members of the component is sent to the Association's Public Relations Department for informational purposes.

The Association's address may be imprinted on or affixed to only printed public relations and public information materials that the Association has agreed to distribute for sections, at cost to those sections, provided that:

*1. The Association's address appears only as a part of the statement "Distributed by the American Physical Therapy Association, 1156 15th Street, N.W. Washington, D.C., 20005," and
2. any such printed material is produced and furnished by the section, and
3. the sale price, if any, for single and multiple copies of such printed material is determined by the section, and

---

*Any such materials must contain the statement if they are to be distributed by the Association.

4. any such printed material does not include newsletters or other periodicals, and

5. the governing body of the section agrees to pay the Association, at a rate determined by the Association, for the services of storing, handling, shipping, and accounting for such printed materials.

Individual members may not display the Association insignia in advertisement of their professional services.

Components and individual members having inquiries about the use of the Association's insignia, name and address not covered in this policy should direct their inquiries to the Executive Director of the American Physical Therapy Association.

Source: Courtesy of The American Physical Therapy Association, Alexandria, VA.

Logo Examples

Logos designed for various physical therapy clinics are shown in Figure 4-1. These logos illustrate a variety of strengths. Many thanks to the physical therapists who graciously allowed their logos to be used in this book. These logos may not be copied or used by anyone other than the organization for whom they were designed.

- The logo for Rehabilitation Services, Ltd., is an easily identified symbol (Figure 4-1A). The person is reaching up, which sends a positive, healthy message. The logo transfers well to other promotional pieces, such as the business card, referral pad, letterhead, and patient information brochure.

- Big Sky Physical Therapy P.C. has a simple, easily identifiable logo (Figure 4-1B). As the mountains are representative of Montana, the logo matches the clinic's name and location. The lines to the right of the mountains express forward movement. The use of blue and eggshell carry the message of health care providers.

- In the logo designed for Duffy & Runyan, the symbol of the hands is combined with the name of the organization (Figure 4-1C). The hands in the shape of a heart express a hands-on, caring attitude, and the use of the last names of the partners as part of the logo expresses personalized service. This logo transfers well to other promotional pieces.

- The hands, representing the personal touch and a caring attitude, are the primary feature of the logo designed for Watrous Physical Therapy (Figure 4-1D). The use of the practitioner's name as part of the clinic name further personalizes this logo. The triangle is a strong and memorable shape, and its use makes this logo similar to that of the American Physical Therapy Association. The triangle points to the words *physical therapy,* which brings the eye to those words.

- The logo of Therex Physical Therapy has an easily identifiable, easy-to-read image (Figure 4-1E). The logo depicts a stylized mountain peak representative of the state of Colorado. The direction of the arrow is upward—symbolic of the progress and movement toward the attainment of goals and peak performance. The logo transfers nicely to other promotional pieces, including the business card, note card, referral pad, and even a Christmas card.
- Somerset Physical Therapy Services has a simple and conservative logo with blue lettering on grey stationery (Figure 4-1F). The use of the APTA's symbol with the word *member* underneath aligns the clinic with traditional values and professional respectability. This logo transfers readily to other promotional forms.
- The simple logo of Grove-Anderson Physical Therapy tells the story of a person getting up (Figure 4-1G). Without words, it leaves the impression that this clinic will get a person going if he or she is down. The logo transfers easily to other promotional pieces.
- The red on grey color combination of the logo used by Burch, Rhoads & Loomis is strong and gives a corporate look to the logo of this multiclinic organization (Figure 4-1H). The use of the names of the original founders in the clinic name personalizes the service. This logo transfers well to other promotional pieces.
- The initials of National Therapeutic Systems, Inc., stylized into a logo is an effective memory jogger for name recognition (Figure 4-1I). This logo will carry through nicely onto promotional materials.
- The graphic design of Wayzata Physical Therapy's logo illustrates the purpose of the business and, therefore, will be remembered (Figure 4-1J). The green print on the eggshell paper represents life. The clinic is named after the town, which affiliates it with the community. The one-on-one care depicted in the logo, combined with the modern and progressive typeface, gives the observer an accurate impression of this clinic at a glance.
- The logo for Carolina Physical Therapy combines the symbol with the practice name in a way that is easy to read (Figure 4-1K). The inner triangle with stripes provides a strong symbol with an expression of forward movement. The use of the two colors green and blue represents life and health.
- The graphic design of the stylized person reaching upward in the logo for Rehabilitation Associates, P.C., combined with the word *rehabilitation* in the name, tells the reader at a glance that this is a business dealing with people (Figure 4-1L). Carrying the first letters of the two words in the name forward into the graphic design reinforces the name. The use of navy blue lettering on grey stock gives a professional, health care image.

REHABILITATION SERVICES, LTD.

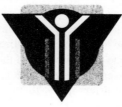

A

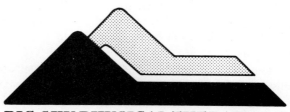

B   **BIG SKY PHYSICAL THERAPY P.C.**

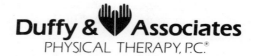

C

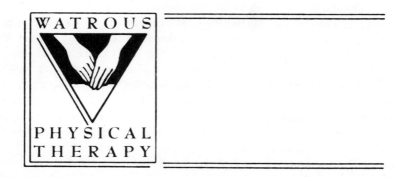

D

Figure 4-1 Logos Designed for Physical Therapy Clinics. **A,** *Source:* Designed by Business Directions, A Marketing and Advertising Firm, Lafayette, Louisiana, for Rehabilitation Services, Ltd., Eunice, Louisiana; **B,** *Source:* Courtesy of Big Sky Physical Therapy P.C., Kalispell, Montana; **C,** *Source:* Courtesy of Duffy & Runyan Physical Therapy, P.C., Des Moines, Iowa; **D,** *Source:* Courtesy of Watrous Physical Therapy, Princeton Junction, New Jersey;

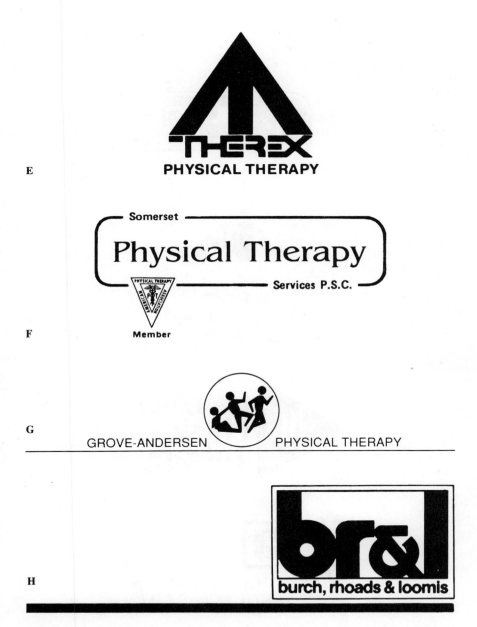

Figure 4-1 continued E, *Source:* Courtesy of Therex Physical Therapy, Littleton, Colorado; **F,** *Source:* Courtesy of Somerset Physical Therapy Services P.S.C., Somerset, Kentucky; **G,** *Source:* Courtesy of Grove-Andersen Physical Therapy, Vallejo, California; **H,** *Source:* Courtesy of Burch, Rhoads & Loomis, Baltimore, Maryland;

continues

I

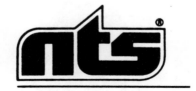

J

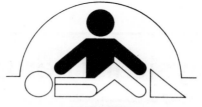

K

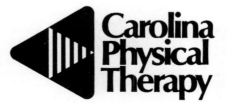

L

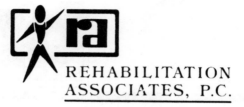

Figure 4-1 continued I, *Source:* Courtesy of National Therapeutic Systems, Inc., Westchester, Illinois; **J,** *Source:* Courtesy of Wayzata Physical Therapy Center, Inc., Plymouth, Minnesota; **K,** *Source:* Courtesy of Carolina Physical Therapy, Hickory, North Carolina; **L,** *Source:* Courtesy of Rehabilitation Associates, P.C., Tucson, Arizona.

NEWSLETTERS

Many physical therapy clinics produce newsletters periodically to keep their target markets informed about special features or services at their clinics. Newsletters are an extremely effective means of public relations, as they present information about the clinic in its therapists' own words, thereby promoting the message that they want to put forward to the exact target population that they choose. Newsletters inform the target market about new services and equipment, professional appointments, accomplishments, and service benefits. Newsletters are most commonly targeted to physicians, consumers, or the organization's employees, although they can be designed for any large target group.

Newsletters can be used as a marketing technique to bring the target market through almost any of the nine steps of the hierarchy of effects (see Chapter 1). A newsletter can be designed to introduce the clinic, explain its benefits, establish interest in its services, promote the decision to purchase new equipment, and stimulate repeat use of the clinic. It must be written specifically with the target market and market plan strategy in mind, however. Used properly, newsletters can benefit a clinic tangibly in terms of improved image, increased visibility, and increased familiarity with the product in the target market.

Benefits of Newsletters

Newsletters excel as promotional tools for many reasons. Primary among these reasons is the clinic staff's control of content, design, production, and distribution; as a result of this control, the newsletter speaks specifically for the clinic that produces it (Exhibit 4-3). This control is a major advantage over other forms of promotion, such as interviews and newspaper articles; in these cases, another person manipulates the clinic's ultimate message.

Therapists' complete control over article content also gives them the opportunity to present their philosophy and point of view in their own words. The message in the newsletter can be personalized so that it brings to the reader a better understanding of the clinic's services. A newsletter reaches *all* members of a specific target market regularly, thus ensuring that the clinic's name, logo, image,

---

Exhibit 4-3 Newsletter Benefits

• Content control	• Personalized message
• Design control	• Targeted reach
• Production and distribution control	• Information approach easily accepted

and identity are frequently in front of the target market, which will promote name recognition and image. This repetitive exposure to the clinic's message helps to establish and maintain referral relationships.

A newsletter is educational, as it contains information of interest to the reader. This educational approach toward marketing is perceived by the reader as informative and helpful. Because it immediately rewards the reader, it may meet with less resistance than do paid advertising and personal selling.

Newsletter Contents

Every newsletter should display prominently the name of the newsletter and the sponsoring organization, in this case, the name of the clinic. If possible, the clinic colors and logo should be used. The address and telephone number must also be included on the newsletter (Exhibit 4-4). Some include a statement about subscription procedures and costs, if any. Additionally, many organizations like to put a short philosophy statement near the heading. For example, the *New York Times* subheading states, "All the News That Is Fit To Print." The clinic's hours of operation and areas of specialty may also be included on the newsletter.

Articles make up most of the newsletter. These articles should be sufficiently brief and concise to ensure some white space and readability. Because "a picture is worth a thousand words," photographs or graphic representations may bring points home. Most newsletters use black and white photographs; the closer the photographer to the subject, the clearer the picture and the greater its reproducibility. Although hiring a graphic artist can be costly, do-it-yourself graphic representations may reduce the professional look of a newsletter. Clip art graphics are generic drawings that have been previously designed and can be purchased in books. Clip art graphics may be used by anyone. Several very good health care clip art books are on the market that can enhance the look of a clinic's newsletter without substantially increasing the clinic's budget. Copyright laws protect graphics, however, so it is necessary to obtain written permission to reprint any graphics. Also, the source should be credited underneath the graphic or at the end of the article.

Exhibit 4-4 Newsletter Contents

- Organization's name, telephone number, address, and hours of operation
- Subscription information
- Philosophy statement
- Articles
- Photographs or graphic representations

Newsletter Format

Newsletters are designed in many sizes, shapes, and colors. A small newsletter in which only one or two ideas are discussed may be typed on a word processor and printed on a single sheet of paper that folds over itself into a self-mailer. Legal size paper works well for this. A larger organization may choose to work with a graphic designer and printing house to create the newsletter. Such a newsletter may resemble a concise one- or two-color newspaper with four to eight pages; it may be mailed in an envelope or brown strip cover. A magazine-type newsletter may be printed on glossy paper using a four-color printing process. Various grades of paper stock may be used. Clearly, the shape and form of newsletters may vary greatly, but even the smallest and most inexpensive newsletter can be attractive, informative, and effective.

Target Market

In choosing which style of newsletter to produce, it is first necessary to determine the target market to be addressed. It is the rare newsletter that is of equal interest to physicians, consumers, and employees. Physicians are interested in a physical therapist's areas of expertise, waiting list (if any), reporting system, and new techniques. Consumers are interested in the clinic's payment policy, waiting time, and treatment outcome. Although similar articles may appear in newsletters for both groups, the tone and slant should differ. For example, an article written to inform physicians about the clinic's recently purchased isokinetic equipment would highlight appropriate patient referral diagnoses and the function of the equipment from a physiological perspective, with quotes and references to research and published articles. A similar article for consumers would emphasize the reduced length of treatment resulting from early physical therapy intervention and its success with professional athletes. A newsletter for employees should include information about the scheduling of in-service educational sessions, upcoming special events, promotions, changes in policies or procedures, and employee benefits.

If the target audience is comprised of fewer than fifty potential readers, the time and cost of producing a newsletter may not be justifiable. In such a case, it may be preferable simply to send a letter with the information to be communicated; a direct mail letter from the clinic's president or director would be appropriate.

The contents of the newsletter should be congruent with the expectations of the target audience. Medical jargon should be avoided in a newsletter for consumers. For example, the word *modality* holds no meaning for patients. It is important to know what will interest the readers and what they should know about the clinic, as well as how much information to give them. Only a knowledge of readers' attitudes, their problems, and their interests ensures the newsletter's readability.

Once the targeted group for the newsletter has been identified, the clinic's strategic marketing plan should be reviewed to determine which marketing goals will be addressed by means of this marketing tool. Articles written for different marketing goals take different slants. For example, in a newsletter intended for a targeted physician public that is unaware of the clinic's existence as in step 1 of the hierarchy of effects (see Chapter 1), the articles should introduce the basic benefits of the clinic. If the purpose of the newsletter is to encourage repeat use (step 8), however, the articles may note awards and educational seminars attended and given by your professional staff. Articles that focus on the information needs of the selected target market enhance the effectiveness of the newsletter as a marketing tool (Exhibit 4-5).

Newsletter Development

In order to develop and evaluate an effective newsletter that will coordinate with the organization's mission and accomplish its marketing goals, it is necessary to begin with market research. (See Exhibit 3-3 for brainstorming exercise with your staff on clinic image.)

A survey should be sent to a random selection of the target market with a self-addressed, stamped return envelope. Although survey questions may vary with the target market, the general categories of questions should include demographics, clinic characteristics, and educational interests (Exhibit 4-6). If the return rate is

---

Exhibit 4-5 Determining the Target Market and Its Information Needs

1. Who will receive the newsletter?

   ☐ Physicians   ☐ Industry
   ☐ Consumers   ☐ Employees
   ☐ Insurance Companies

2. Will the target market be one or a combination of the above?

   _____   _____

3. For *this* issue of the newsletter, where is the target market in the hierarchy of effects?

   ☐ 1 Unawareness   ☐ 6 Decision
   ☐ 2 Awareness   ☐ 7 Satisfaction
   ☐ 3 Understanding   ☐ 8 Repeat use
   ☐ 4 Familiarity   ☐ 9 Recommendation
   ☐ 5 Interest

Exhibit 4-6 Newsletter Audience Survey

Dear Doctor _____:

Your comments about our newsletter are important to us so that it can continue to improve our services. We appreciate your completing the enclosed survey and returning it in the self-addressed, stamped envelope.

1. Demographics
   - _____ Age
   - _____ Sex
   - _____ Occupation/Specialty
2. What would you like to know about our clinic?
   - _____ Location
   - _____ Hours
   - _____ Payment policy
   - _____ Specialties
   - _____ Staff expertise
   - _____ Equipment
3. Rank the type of articles that interest you the most.
   - _____ Case study
   - _____ New techniques
   - _____ Prevention
   - _____ Exercise protocols
   - _____ Information about staff

---

greater than 20 percent, the results may be considered valid, and the suggestions and recommendations found on the survey should be followed.

Articles

Ideas for articles can come from several sources (Exhibit 4-7). Many clinic directors keep a folder in which to put ideas whenever they run across suitable ones so that they will never be at a loss for article ideas. Newspapers contain many articles pertaining to physical therapy, such as those on fitness or exercise, disability management, and even insurance claims reimbursement, that may deserve space in a clinic's newsletter. An article may be reprinted in the newsletter with permission from the original publisher, or a new article may be written to state the clinic staff's opinion as it relates to the news article. Health and sports magazines also have many articles that relate to physical therapy.

The topics of interest to the public can often be identified from current health magazines. Additionally, APTA publications, such as *Progress Report, The Component Bulletin*, and even *Physical Therapy Journal* and *Clinical Management*, can be sources of ideas. The various brochures that the APTA has produced also contain excellent sources of information and ideas for newsletters. Physicians

Exhibit 4-7 Newsletter Articles

- Where to find ideas for articles:
  1. Newspapers
  2. Magazines
  3. Reprints
  4. APTA Publications
  5. Target markets
- How to write articles:
  1. Audience perspective
  2. Content brevity
  3. Main points first
  4. Interviews
  5. Keep newsletter goals in mind
- What is newsworthy:
  1. New information
  2. Human interest
  3. Controversy
- Emphasize your differential advantage

and patients may also have suggestions. Interviews are often of interest to a target market, particularly if they are with an expert physical therapist, a member of the target market, or an outside expert discussing an inside problem. Interviews are easy to read, and they capture people's attention.

In writing the articles, it is necessary constantly to keep in mind the members of the target audience and to think from their perspective. The article should be brief and to the point. Major points should be highlighted. The main point of the article should always appear in the first sentence, as many people may skim the newsletter and read only the first sentence. Following the main point of the article, support statements should be listed.

It is important to keep in mind the purpose of the message, as well as the clinic image to be presented through the article and the goal of this particular marketing effort. Is this newsletter intended simply to increase the awareness of the clinic within the target market, to increase referrals, or simply to provide information to the target market? The type of message and its wording will depend on the purpose of the particular newsletter and its role within the marketing plan.

Because the publication is a *newsletter*, articles should deal with new information, human interest, or controversy. "New" information may not necessarily be new to physical therapists, but it will be new to the target market. For example, the benefits of a neurodevelopmental approach in the treatment of upper motor neuron dysfunction is definitely not new information to physical therapists, but it will be new information to the parents who have recently been told that their young child has cerebral palsy. Human interest has always been considered newsworthy. An article about a patient is a human interest story, particularly if the patient is well-known, such as a professional athlete; however, the use of a patient story requires the permission of the patient. Controversy is also considered news. For example, a newsletter article on the controversy over the use of lumbar flexion exercises versus the use of extension exercises, or a combination of both, would be appropriate.

Creativity is the watchword in designing and developing a newsletter in terms of the way that it is folded, the number of pages, its color design, and its overall appearance. It is important to use white space wisely. A newsletter that is filled with solid print is less likely to be read than one that is laid out with eye-catching white space and contrasting graphics. Newsletters received at the clinic should be examined with a critical eye to determine which ones are more readable than others, and some of the best features can be incorporated into the clinic's newsletter.

In general, a newsletter should emphasize the clinic's differential advantage, the features that make it special and different from the competition. It is often helpful to ask a layperson to read the articles for interest and to determine the effectiveness of the manner in which the differential advantage is presented.

Use of Consultants

Once the newsletter articles have been written, it may be wise to contact a consultant. Many printers can provide valuable assistance in the production of a newsletter. For a glossier look, a graphic artist or agency may be hired to produce the newsletter. An editor may be hired to edit the copy. Any of these consultants can make recommendations about the general format.

Newsletters are usually one to four pages in length. A newsletter can be folded like a newspaper or just folded into itself. Of course, an 8½ by 11 inch page can be folded to fit nicely into an envelope. Another option is to use a single 8½ by 11 inch page and fold it over to make it a self-mailer. This eliminates the need for an envelope, but makes it necessary to leave space for the return address and the mailing address, thus reducing the amount of copy space.

When the format has been selected, the newsletter can be reproduced by photocopying or by offset printing. The consultant should be able to help in the preparation of the graphics and layout, as well as to offer suggestions concerning printing and writing style.

Cost

The clinic's first newsletter will be more expensive and require more time than subsequent newsletters, because the graphic designer will need to design the overall format and masthead for the first one. When these decisions have been made, the simple placement of the articles in subsequent newsletters is much less costly. The cost of the initial design and set-up for the newsletter is likely to be between $300 and $800. Mailing or other distribution is an additional cost.

The advent of desktop publishing creates a less expensive alternative to newsletter production through a printing house. As with the traditionally produced newsletter, the first newsletter is the most difficult to produce by means of desk top publishing because the format, heading, and design must be selected and set up for the first time.

Prepared Newsletters

If physical therapists do not wish to produce a newsletter themselves, with or without consultants, but think a newsletter would be beneficial to their marketing efforts, there are several agencies that produce physical therapy newsletters. They will put the clinic's name on the masthead. They will do everything from writing the articles to printing and mailing the newsletters. Most of these prepared newsletters are targeted to patients.

Marketing Uses of the Newsletter

In order to receive a positive return on the investment of time and money, the newsletter needs to be incorporated into the marketing plan. A newsletter is most often used as a direct mailer to the target market. It can be a subtle, but persuasive, way to put the clinic's name in front of the target market, thus establishing name recognition. Physical therapy clinics can also use newsletters to

- maintain interest in the clinic, reminding the target audience that the clinic continues to provide professional quality services.
- stimulate interest in the target audience through various articles.
- improve the familiarity of the target audience with the various aspects of the clinic.
- educate the target public concerning the clinic's specialty. Most people have only a very superficial knowledge of physical therapy and can benefit from additional information.
- stimulate word-of-mouth promotion by leaving it in the reception area for patients to take home. They can also be encouraged to give the newsletter to their friends to read.

A newsletter can be helpful on a sales call as a leave-behind piece to remind the prospect of the clinic's business and to make the product, which is a service product, more tangible. A newsletter can also be used as a public lecture handout to emphasize the staff's professionalism and, again, to increase the tangibility of the clinic's services. A special edition of the newsletter can be included as an introductory piece in the marketing packet. Copies of the newsletter can be taken to health fairs and other public events where people pick up information and brochures.

Newsletter Evaluation

Market research techniques can be used to evaluate the newsletter's effectiveness (Exhibit 4-8). After substantial time, effort, and money have been invested to create, distribute, and use a newsletter, it is only logical to evaluate its effectiveness. Such an evaluation should focus on the marketing purpose of the newsletter. If the purpose was to introduce the clinic's name, a sample of those who received

---

Exhibit 4-8 Target Market Research

1. Determine your target market.
   - Who will receive the Newsletter? (physicians, consumers, insurance companies, industry employees)
   - Will the target market be one or a combination of the above?

2. Where is your target market in the Hierarchy of Effects?

3. What type of news is appropriate for this target market?

4. Review your strategic marketing plan and list the marketing goals you will address with your newsletter.

5. List the three adjectives that best describe your clinic.
   1.
   2.
   3.
6. List the results of your audience survey.

7. Review article file for ideas.

8. List your plans to market your newsletter.

the newsletter can be called to determine name recognition. If the purpose was to familiarize the target market with clinic benefits, a similar telephone survey can be conducted to ask questions specifically related to the benefits highlighted in the newsletter. Alternatively, the same survey that was sent to the target market before the newsletter was produced may be sent to determine changed or static interest. If the purpose of the newsletter was to increase referrals, a computer can be used to track referral patterns in the target market to whom the newsletter was sent.

The results of the evaluation process are helpful in designing future marketing efforts. It may be discovered that newsletters are effective in increasing repeat business, but ineffective in introducing the clinic's name and logo. If this is true, future newsletters should be sent to individuals who are already familiar with the clinic. Nevertheless, it is imperative to establish a tool to evaluate the effectiveness of this project.

Example of a Newsletter

Exhibit 4-9 is a generic newsletter that provides new and interesting information to the health care consumer. It can be customized with a clinic's own logo, name, address, and telephone number.

BROCHURES

A brochure is a pamphlet or booklet designed to provide information. For a physical therapy clinic, an informational brochure about its service features should be one of the first marketing tools created after its mission, target market, position, and image have been determined. Brochures are excellent introductory pieces to use when the target market is in step 1 of the hierarchy of effects (i.e., when the target market is unaware of the clinic's existence). An informational brochure can be used at almost any of the nine steps to reinforce the clinic's message and image, however. The benefits of brochures are listed in Exhibit 4-10.

The biggest pitfall in designing and developing a brochure is to do so because "everyone says that in order to market your clinic you need to have a brochure." The only reason ever to design and develop a brochure for a clinic is to achieve specific objectives and goals. Most physical therapy clinics need a brochure because of the diverse opportunities for use. First, however, it is essential to examine the organization's mission statement, to identify the target audience, and to determine the method of distribution. Those people involved in designing and developing brochures know horror stories of thousands of dollars spent on a brochure that no one ever used because it was obsolete or the program that it promoted changed before the brochure was even distributed.

Exhibit 4-9 Example of a Newsletter

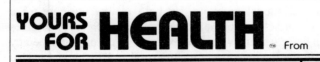

YOURS FOR HEALTH... From

THE OCCASIONAL GARDENER
Weeding Out Back Problems

When Contrary Mary was asked how here garden grew, she never mentioned spading, weeding, or carrying buckets. In short, she didn't relate "putting her back" into her work.

That's great, because a major cause of low back pain is the result of misusing back muscles.

This article is a physical labor trip through garden care, providing tips for good body mechanics. We suggest how you, too, can keep your back out of work.

Preparing the Soil

A fork or spade in hand, your task is to turn over the soil. Plunge the tool into the ground using the foot as extra weight. When it reaches a depth of 8 inches, push down on the handle to loosen the soil. Do this by bending at the knees primarily.

In lifting the soil to turn it slightly or throw it onto a pile, **step**—ie, move your foot toward the throwing site. For example, you want to throw dirt into a wheelbarrow on your left. First bend at the knees. Shovel up the dirt. Lift by straightening your knees. Move your left foot toward the wheelbarrow. Then put the dirt in. **Don't twist.**

When you break up clods of soil with a spade, bend and straighten knees to supply power. Stand right over the dirt balls and smash them by bringing the spade down as though it were a pole you were driving into the ground.

Use your legs to rake or hoe; avoid twisting at the waist.

Planting & Weeding

Most likely *only* well-conditioned athletes are flexible enough to bend at the waist with unbended knees to plant a garden without incurring sacroiliac or lumbosacral problems, such as sciatica.

So, if bending at the waist is comfortable for you, do so with bent knees. Otherwise, squatting or kneeling are fine. (Kneel on a rolled up blanket or pad to avoid irritating the inner lining of your knee that causes painful swelling—Housemaid's knee or *tenosynovitis.*)

Lifting & Carrying:
Wheelbarrows & Buckets

Pick up the wheelbarrow handles by first bending the knees, then straightening. **Do not bend at the waist and straighten to lift.**

To push the wheelbarrow, keep knees slightly bent so the weight remains primarily on the thighs rather than on the low back.

To dump the load, pushing forward is probably less stressful on the body than dumping to the side. Either way, dump the load by moving your foot toward the direction of the dump. Do not twist at the waist or keep your feet stationary.

Pick up loaded buckets by bending and straightening your knees. (Alternate carrying in different hands. This helps relieve stress on elbows, which otherwise could result in "tennis elbow" type problems.) It is better to carry two loaded buckets than one to prevent an uneven stress from developing on one side of your back. If the weight of one load is so heavy that your back is

Featured in this Issue:

Gardening & Back Problems

Food Cravings

Food & Health Tips

Current Research

Review

twisted to one side, you're carrying too much. Divide that load into two buckets or make two trips instead.

Trimming

Makes no difference whether you use a power cutter or manual shears: remember your feet are not set in concrete. Pivot your body by moving your feet as you trim the hedge. Avoid twisting at the waist.

A summary for good body mechanics—whether it be to move furniture, garden, or shovel snow— is to put as much of your load on your legs as

"GARDENER" cont. page 3

Source: Reprinted with permission of Panos Communications, Ltd., Tequesta, Florida.

Exhibit 4-10 Benefits of Brochures

- Quality Enhancer
- Memory Jogger
- Educational Reinforcer
- Image Promoter
- Referral Stimulator

Benefits of a Brochure

An informational or educational brochure can be a quality attribute for a physical therapy department, clinic, or home care practice. Because it gives patients and/or potential referral sources tangible evidence of the physical therapy service, a brochure reinforces the message of quality service. Brochures can also reiterate information that therapists have imparted during treatment sessions, which helps patients to remember the message correctly.

Brochures are an excellent and time-honored way to introduce a clinic's logo and image to target markets. Brochures can focus on the special features of a clinic's service, such as the education and training of its staff and the accessibility of its location. A brochure of this type can help current patients remember and explain the details of the clinic's service to family, friends, and other medical personnel. Brochures such as this can also be given to potential referral sources, such as physicians, social workers, or nurses.

Brochures are also an educational reinforcement for patients who have common medical conditions and for patients who need information on preventive care. If the physical therapists at the clinic frequently teach transfer techniques to families, a brochure that describes the "how-to's" and "do's and don'ts" of transfers can be helpful for families to use at home as a supplement to the personal instruction session(s). Other ideas for useful educational brochures are

- prevention of re-injury
- activities of daily living, common examples
- what to expect from physical therapy
- how to file insurance claims
- specific basic exercises for selected joints or diseases

A good brochure promotes and reinforces the clinic's image. As used in marketing, it may be the clinic's first impression on the target audience. Therefore, all design features, such as the type of paper stock, print style, and graphics, should reflect the clinic's true image. Any incongruence between promotional materials and actual service will significantly reduce patient satisfaction. If the clinic is a low-budget facility with cramped space and only basic technological equipment, but has experienced therapists with advanced manual skills who spend a significant amount of time with each patient, a fancy and expensive brochure would be out of place. More appropriate would be the use of a good, but not the best, quality stock, with a simple, clear design and a focus on wording that describes and promotes therapist expertise.

When the brochure is designed to match the clinic's quality features and is used frequently in marketing efforts, it will encourage referrals. Sent as a direct mailer or given out at the time of a lecture or sales call, it can be just the reminder needed to stimulate a referral. Even referral sources who are familiar with the clinic may be surprised at some of the benefits highlighted in the brochure and, thus, may send additional referrals.

Brochure Contents

The target market determines the appropriate contents of a brochure. The brochure may be written to address past, present, and/or new target markets to update or inform them of the clinic's services. The brochure may be directed toward physicians, patients, or industry.

It is difficult for a brochure to be all things for all target markets. The information desired by physicians may be very different from that desired by patients, for example. A brochure for physicians may highlight the highly sophisticated equipment in the clinic and the scheduling of appointments for their patients within twenty-four hours of referral. The brochure can also list the schools and accomplishments of individual staff members. In contrast, potential patients are more interested in treatment outcomes, practice location, costs, and hours of operation.

In order to make a brochure more versatile, it could have a slot in a back flap into which inserts can be placed. For example, each insert could have a different physical therapist's picture and credentials so that the brochure would be individualized and personalized when a physical therapist goes on a sales call. Inserts that highlight special programs could be used to target particular audiences. Such inserts could focus on sports medicine, geriatric, or health injury prevention programs.

Unless the brochure is for a new high-visibility, high-budget clinic or program and there is no doubt that market research has accurately defined the proper content and extent of the program, it is unwise to spend a great deal of money on designing an expensive brochure initially. The program may change over time, particularly in the first year or two, and the expensive brochure is likely to be obsolete. A satisfactory brochure that can be copied at the printer on a very small budget can be designed and developed in-house to meet the initial needs for a new clinic or program. Care must be taken to ensure that a brochure produced in-house does not look amateurish and is not difficult to read, however, as the image that it projects will be less professional.

The common elements of a general brochure that focuses on the clinic's quality aspects include the clinic's name, telephone number, address, logo, specialties, equipment, and differential advantage. (See Exhibit 4-11 for additional items to be included on a brochure's contents.) The clinic's name, address, and telephone number should be displayed in a prominent location. The logo, if available, should

Exhibit 4-11 Brochure Content

A brochure should include the following:

- Organization name
- Principle staff and staff biographies
- Address
- Telephone number
- Map
- Logo in identifying color(s)
- Mission statement
- Philosophy
- Services and programs
  —Specialties and areas of expertise
  —Equipment (especially unique equipment such as a pool or isokinetic equipment)
- Modalities
- Payment policy
- Differential advantage

---

be included, and the colors chosen previously for the clinic's stationery should be used. Many clinics include their mission statement and/or philosophy of service. A map may also be helpful. If the organization is fairly small, staff biographies help to personalize the message. Programs and special services that differentiate the clinic from its competition may be listed. Some clinics like to list modalities that are offered at the clinic. Although physicians may respond well to a listing of modalities, some patients may not understand the meaning of modalities in terms of treatment outcome. In some cases, it is wise to list payment policy on the brochure.

Brochure Format

Once plans have been made for the use of the brochure during the next year in marketing efforts, marketing priorities should be established. If the brochure is to be distributed primarily through the mail, a single or dual fold brochure that will fit into an envelope may help to control mailing costs. If the brochure is to be used primarily in sales calls and as handouts, the designer can be more creative in the number of folds and weight of paper.

Brochure Development

In beginning to plan a brochure, the first step is to do some homework in the form of market research. It is essential to decide on the image to be projected through the brochure and to carry this image through in the color and stock of paper, the type of print, the writing style, and the use of white space. The only way to determine what the target audience expects from the clinic's services and what they want to know from the brochure is to ask them in survey form, either a telephone survey or a written survey. By surveying the target market, it is possible to determine what differential advantages are important (Exhibit 4-12).

In writing the brochure copy, comments should be personalized. If the writer imagines himself or herself sitting down and talking to one member of the target market, the brochure will sound warm and friendly. It is important to remember that a brochure is not a scientific paper or a term paper. It is a tool for communication with the target market.

Before designing the clinic's brochure, it is helpful to examine at least twenty brochures from other health care agencies, both local and national, and another ten brochures that have been produced commercially for other types of products. Creative ideas may result from looking through the various brochures and determining what image they are trying to project, whether they actually reach their proposed audience, and what the color and type of paper does. For example, bright colors and glossy paper suggest a contemporary image, while subdued colors and textured paper project a traditional image. The size and the number of folds, the type of print, and the use of graphics, including pictures and sketches, should also be examined. A form such as that shown in Exhibit 4-13 may be used to record the impressions made by these brochures.

Once therapists at the clinic have reviewed carefully all the brochures collected, they can be creative in designing the clinic's brochure by adding their own personal touches. They can do something that no one else in the area is doing. For example, glossy paper may be used if no one else is using it in a brochure. The brochure could be folded differently; it could be made larger or smaller. Inserts or

---

Exhibit 4-12 Brochure Audience Survey

Dear Doctor _____:

Your comments about our brochures are important to us so that we can continue to improve our services. We appreciate your completing the enclosed survey and returning it in the self-addressed, stamped envelope.

Rank the following items as important for you from physical therapy:

_____ Location	_____ Technology
_____ Hours	_____ Payment policy
_____ Cost	_____ Expertise
_____ Experience	_____ Equipment
_____ Recommendation	

Exhibit 4-13 Evaluation of Competitors' Brochures

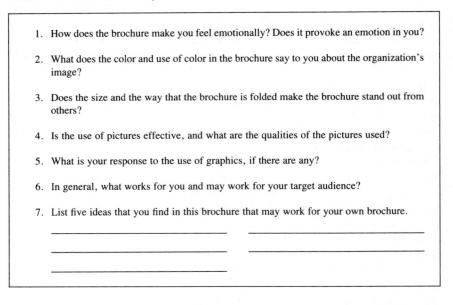

1. How does the brochure make you feel emotionally? Does it provoke an emotion in you?

2. What does the color and use of color in the brochure say to you about the organization's image?

3. Does the size and the way that the brochure is folded make the brochure stand out from others?

4. Is the use of pictures effective, and what are the qualities of the pictures used?

5. What is your response to the use of graphics, if there are any?

6. In general, what works for you and may work for your target audience?

7. List five ideas that you find in this brochure that may work for your own brochure.

combinations of white space and print could be unusual. The life expectancy of a brochure varies, depending on the changing external and internal environment. As consumer expectations change and as staff members and internal programs change, the brochure will need to be updated.

Use of Consultants

At this point, it is time to contact a graphic designer (see section on Logos) and, possibly, a health care writer if there will be a significant amount of prose in the brochure. The graphic designer will provide essentially the same services in designing the brochure as in designing the logo. It is wise to obtain three or more proposals from area consultants. They will vary surprisingly, and the clinic staff will learn something from each proposal.

Health care brochures previously created by the consultant or firm should be reviewed, if possible. Former clients given as references should be asked if the consultants met their deadlines, stayed within budget, and were generally helpful during the production process. Often, additional costs are incurred for additional samples. Firms and consultants experienced in designing health care brochures are sensitive to wording and design that is acceptable to the clinic's target market.

The consultant will provide assistance in deciding on the general format of the brochure, the use of the clinic's logo on the brochure, colors, typeface, and stock of paper. A good printer can offer advice about the image that various paper and print colors and color combinations will create. Blues and greens are cool, while browns and reds are warm. Beige and blue are more traditional health care colors, while burgundy and teal depict a more progressive image.

Costs

Brochures produced in-house, typed on a word processor, and photocopied on white or colored paper, have indirect costs of staff time for writing, editing, layout, and proofing, in addition to typist time and copier usage. Direct costs are those of the paper and mailing. This is still the least expensive way to produce a brochure, however, as it costs from $100 to $200. Brochures produced this way can state the message clearly and function as effective marketing tools. If your content is well written, concise, and directed specifically to the target market, it can be well received. It demonstrates a concern for information distribution rather than a flashy appearance. If the clinic emphasizes cost containment or provides free and discounted care to the poor or indigent, this brochure format corresponds with its overall image. As the clinic grows, the brochure budget may allow for professional editing and graphic design, but the production process should be kept economical.

A typical one- or two-fold health services brochure produced with the assistance of a good printer can cost $1,000 to $6,000, or $0.75 to $1.50 per brochure, assuming that the logo has already been designed. Adding one or two colors to a brochure can enhance its readability and, thus, improve it as a communications tool. Color photographs in the brochure require a four-color printing process, and the brochure cost jumps considerably. This cost may be worth it, however, if color photographs will personalize the clinic's service for the reader. Professionally produced brochures such as this can cost between $2,000 and $5,000, depending on the number of colors used, number of pages, number of brochures printed and rates of the printer.

Marketing Uses of the Brochure

Although most physical therapists will benefit from designing a brochure to promote their differential advantages, two phases must occur first. First, they must know their target market. Second, they must know in which marketing efforts they plan to use the brochure. Knowledge of these two factors will influence the design, layout, graphics, and even language used. For example, a brochure geared to the general public would use terms like *neck* and *low back*; the terms *cervical* and *lumbar* would be substituted in a physician-targeted brochure. Although regular typeface would be appropriate for a brochure directed to the general public, larger print is preferable for the over sixty-five age group.

The marketing efforts for which the brochure is created also influence design. Although an oversized brochure of heavy stock may be appropriate and memorable as a lecture handout, a two- or three-fold envelope-sized brochure in medium weight paper stock would be less expensive to produce and distribute as a direct mail piece. Designing a brochure before establishing the strategic marketing plan leaves too many important design decisions to chance.

Brochures are extremely versatile and universal marketing tools. They can effectively promote the clinic when incorporated into the strategic marketing plan for audiences at various stages in the hierarchy of effects. Brochures are sent as a direct mail promotion to stimulate interest, maintain interest, or stimulate word-of-mouth public relations. Used as a handout and leave-behind piece during a sales call, they can help promote a decision to use the therapist's service. They can also serve as handouts at lectures to the community and at health fairs to increase audience exposure to the message. A copy of the brochure can accompany an introductory marketing packet to help explain the clinic's differential advantage. When distributed to current and past patients, brochures can promote word-of-mouth referrals by encouraging distribution among friends and family who may themselves benefit from physical therapy.

Brochure Evaluation

The development of the brochure began with market research, and the cycle ends with market research as well. Now that a brochure has been created specifically for the clinic and has been used in the clinic's marketing efforts, it is time to evaluate its effectiveness.

- Did the brochure increase referrals?
- Did it improve awareness of the clinic?
- Did it educate and increases familiarity of the target market with the clinic?

Brochure effectiveness can be evaluated by tracking referrals through computer data, as well as through follow-up surveys in which the target audience previously surveyed is asked specific questions concerning the effectiveness of the brochure.

Brochure Examples

The following are examples of physical therapy practice brochures produced by physical therapists across the country. They are diverse in their presentation style, from a one-page two fold to a sixteen-page staple binding with staff inserts. Their commonality is the prominent display of the organization's logo throughout. Exhibit 4-14A is a patient information brochure that carries the logo of geometric design throughout as bullets and highlights and thus reinforces the image. White space is used for easy readability. The signatures of clinic owners add a personalized touch. Exhibit 4-14B is a patient information brochure that graphically links muscles and joints with activity and health through the illustration and copy on the front, thus promoting the organization's position. The back of the brochure is dedicated to answering accessibility questions such as location, parking, hours of operation, insurance policies, address and telephone number. The inside copy is brief and easy to read, highlighting the organization's position. Not shown here are program inserts featuring information of interest to special target markets. Exhibit 4-14C is a six page, staple bound glossy stock brochure of the Back School of Atlanta. It is clear and professional leaving the reader with a good understanding of its purpose. The logo appears on each page for reinforcement. The target market of this brochure is physical therapy clinics that may want to purchase the products described.

NEWS RELEASES

Some physical therapy services are of such community interest that they are promoted by the media free of charge. An announcement of such a service through the news release is a good way to get a clinic's name in front of the public without the cost of advertising space. A news release can be sent either to print media (press release) or broadcast media (broadcast release).

A news release should contain information of interest to the public, such as a discussion of new services, an announcement of a special event (e.g., a health fair, lecture, or meeting), or an explanation of a medical fact (e.g., the importance of warm-up and stretching in an overall fitness program). A news release can be an announcement, such as the opening of a particular clinic or service. If a news release is an announcement about a clinic staff member, it should include information of local interest.

Another type of news release involves the impact of current events on a physical therapy clinic. If, for example, an increase in reports of Lyme disease has resulted in an increase in referrals to the clinic for joint pain, a news release about this event may catch a reporter's eye as an item of community interest. Similarly, if therapists at the clinic are treating a number of workers who were injured in a factory accident and the investigation of this incident becomes an ongoing press item, the clinic's response to the event may attract the attention of a reporter for use as an article.

Exhibit 4-14 Examples of Brochures

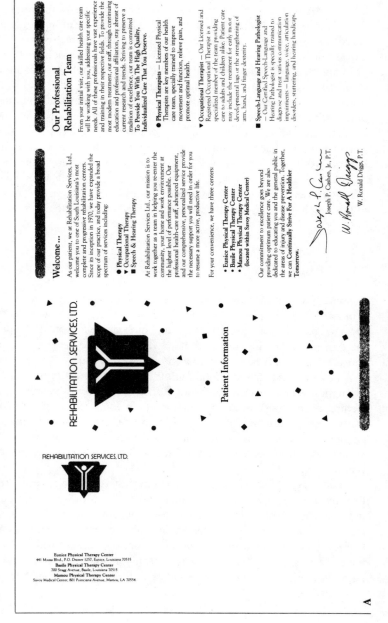

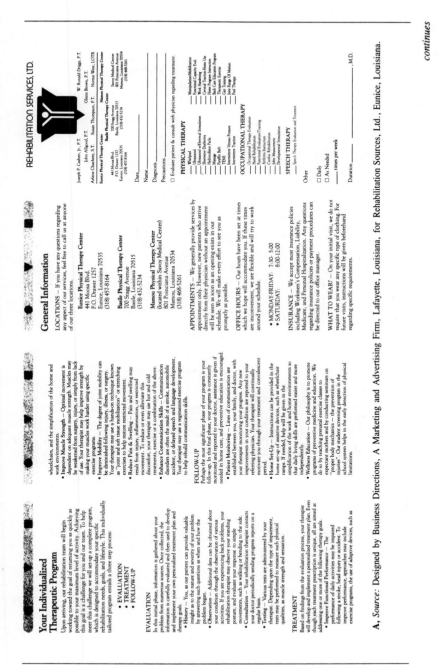

A, *Source:* Designed by Business Directions, A Marketing and Advertising Firm, Lafayette, Louisiana, for Rehabilitation Sources, Ltd., Eunice, Louisiana.

continues

Exhibit 4-14 continued

B

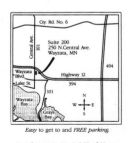

Easy to get to and *FREE parking.*

Appointments: M - F 7:30 - 6:00 pm
Sat. 8:00 - 12:00 noon

We accept private insurers, workers compensation, Medicaid, Medicare, Blue Cross/Blue Shield, and most HMO's, including Aware Gold, Group Health Inc., Physicians Health Plan (PHP), HMO Minnesota, Share and Family Health Network.

State licensed physical therapists.

Wayzata Medical Building
250 North Central Avenue, Suite 200
Wayzata, MN 55391

(612) 473-4972

Wayzata
Physical Therapy
Center, Inc.

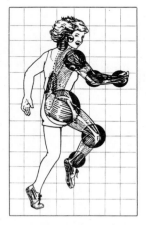

**Dedicated to helping *You*
maintain your active life style.**

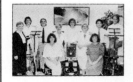

History

The Wayzata Physical Therapy Center and the Sports Clinic have been providing physical therapy in the western suburbs of Minneapolis since 1971. Today the center includes 6 professional therapists on staff with over 70 years of professional experience. The clinic offers general physical therapy treatments to decrease pain, and increase function and mobility so you may return to your active life style. Your therapist treats such problem areas as backs, necks, knees, shoulders, ankles, hands, TMJ, etc. Specific conditions such as sprains, strains, arthritis, spinal/disc problems, and orthopedic and sports related injuries are frequently treated at the Wayzata Physical Therapy Center and Sports Clinic.

We can make a difference in your life style by promoting "Quality" care. A personal approach is taken with every patient to insure individualized treatments with specific goals for each patient.

Services

Our clinic has specialized equipment such as computerized Cybex II+, Fitron, UBE, Orthotron, pulleys and Eagle equipment. We utilize modalities such as electrical stimulation, ultrasound, TENS, whirlpool, traction, iontophoresis, muscle stimulation, heat and ice.

Among all this hi-tech equipment is something more important: *YOU!* Our patients, whether youngsters, athletes or senior citizens, will respond to therapy in a warm, friendly atmosphere with our staff. We spend time listening to you to understand your specific needs.

Minnesota now allows Physical Therapy without a physician's referral. If your condition requires a doctor's attention, we will refer you to your physician. If you don't have one, we can recommend a doctor with expertise for your specific condition. Patients sent to the Wayzata Physical Therapy Center with prescription referrals by doctors will have those orders followed precisely. Close communication with the patient's physician is maintained throughout the treatment.

B, *Source:* Courtesy of Wayzata Physical Therapy Center, Inc., Plymouth, Minnesota.

Exhibit 4-14 continued

C

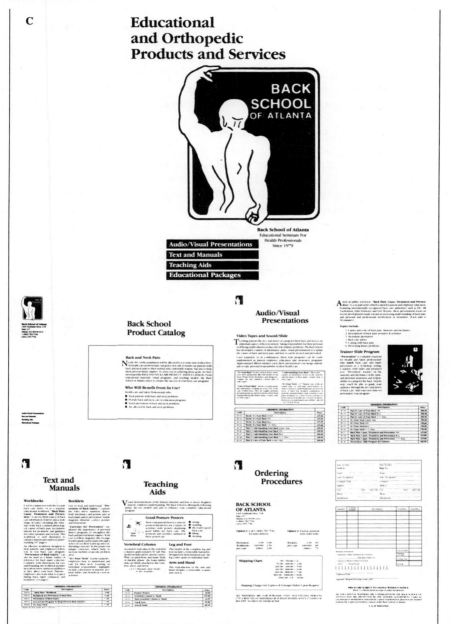

C, *Source:* Courtesy of Back School of Atlanta, Atlanta, Georgia.

News Release Format

A news release should be typed, double spaced on standard size plain paper with 1½-inch margins all around. Text should be typed on only one side of the paper. The copy should begin approximately two inches below the heading so that an editor can insert a different heading if desired. It is preferable for a news release to be one page; if two pages are necessary, "more" should be typed at the center of the bottom of the first page. The news release should end with "end," "# # #," or "30."

Letterhead stationery for the purpose of name recognition may be used in lieu of plain white paper. In either case, the heading must contain the organization's name, address, name of the contact person, and the telephone number. An evening telephone number should also be included, as news reporters often work outside regular business hours. In addition, the intended date of the release should be in the heading. Release may be "immediate," but it may be preferable to put a specific release date several days in advance so that all the media have the opportunity to release the information at the same time, ensuring that no one source receives an advantage.

The headline should summarize the content of the news release. It should be brief, less than one line in length, and written in the active present tense.

The main point of a news release should always be stated in the first sentence, and the major following points should be included in the first paragraph. The remaining paragraphs simply add detail for the summary statement. This arrangement is important, because the person in the news room who scans news releases must make a decision whether to use it based on the first few seconds of reading. Additionally, if the news release must be cut, it will be cut from the bottom up, and this arrangement ensures that the main point of the article remains within the published piece.

At least two people should proofread the news release. It is easy for an author to overlook simple typographical or grammatical errors.

News stories contain answers to the following questions: who, what, where, why, when, and how. A news release should also answer those questions. The sentences should be short and interesting, and they should contain no medical jargon. The writer should imagine that he or she is a typical reader who is not familiar with physical therapy.

Distribution

A news release should be distributed to media that reach the target audience interested in the clinic's message. Reading the local newspaper, listening to local radio stations, and watching local television stations will reveal which ones report on health and what types of articles and releases are currently accepted. Many local newspapers and city magazines have writers and editors with an interest in health and human interest items. Radio and television shows that already feature health experts and tips will be more open to the clinic's news item than are those that historically avoid health news. Shows that emphasize community service are also good targets because of their demonstrated commitment to public well-being.

All media sources that are potential outlets for the clinic's news should be listed. Media personnel information, job titles, and telephone numbers can be obtained locally. A news release can be mailed or faxed to everyone on the identified media source list. A therapist who knows someone on the staff of the newspaper or radio or television station may call that person to discuss the content of a news release and the possibility of its use in that particular medium. A follow-up call is a good method to check that the release has been received, to answer questions, and to encourage coverage. It is helpful to obtain both positive and negative comments so that the next release can better fit that medium's slant on the news. Such a call may also lead to an invitation for an interview, an appearance on a talk show, or further coverage of the therapist's activities. In any case, the therapist should elicit feedback for future releases.

It is essential to be patient and persistent. Media people are extremely busy and do not necessarily inform the originator of what has happened to a news release. They are always looking for news, however, and persistence may pay off. The principle of the hierarchy of effects applies to the media just as it applies to target markets.

If a therapist sends news releases regularly, such as once a month, to the local media, one or two of the releases may catch a reporter's eye, and the therapist may become an expert resource. In time, the reporter may be calling that therapist as an expert for a reaction, interpretation, quotation, or opinion. Exhibit 4-15 is a worksheet for the seven elements in news release production.

Example of News Release

The news release in Exhibit 4-16 was produced by the American Physical Therapy Association (APTA) for distribution and use by the local chapters to promote the profession.

PUBLIC SPEAKING

Speaking before groups of people about physical therapy can effectively establish and position a therapist as an expert in the community. Whether the groups are small or large, speaking before them requires practice and preparation to ensure

Exhibit 4-15 News Release Worksheet

1. Determine audience(s) (target market):

   _____

2. Determine media:

   Print   *Broadcast*
   ☐ Newspaper   ☐ Radio
   ☐ Magazine   ☐ Television

3. List possible media distribution points and contact persons:

   _____   _____

   _____   _____

   _____   _____

4. Determine content:

   ☐ New service/clinic   ☐ Staff news
   ☐ Announcement of special event ☐ Current event
   ☐ Medical news

5. Follow format:

   A. Use 8½ by 11½ inch white paper.
   B. Allow 1½-inch margins all around.
   C. Double-space.
   D. Type only on one side of the paper.
   E. Begin content 2 inches below heading.
   F. Type "end" or "###" at end of release.
   G. Heading includes organization's name, address, telephone number, and name of contact person.
   H. State release date.

6. Determine headline:

   _____

7. Answer the question(s):
   Who, what, where, why, how, and when.

that the message will be delivered in an organized and memorable fashion. The appropriate use of audiovisual aides, such as slides, overhead projectors, and videocassette recorders, can significantly enhance a speech. The selection of the target audience should be based on the potential publicity for the clinic and its specific clientele.

Benefits of Public Speaking

Public speaking by health care professionals is a time-honored tradition and, as a form of marketing, is well accepted both by consumers of health care and by

Exhibit 4-16 News Release Example

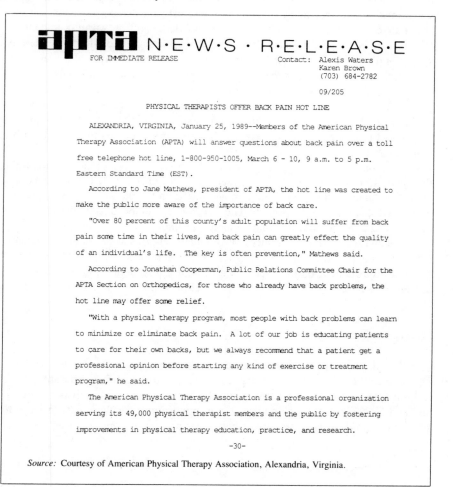

APTA N·E·W·S · R·E·L·E·A·S·E

FOR IMMEDIATE RELEASE

Contact: Alexis Waters
Karen Brown
(703) 684-2782

09/205

PHYSICAL THERAPISTS OFFER BACK PAIN HOT LINE

ALEXANDRIA, VIRGINIA, January 25, 1989--Members of the American Physical Therapy Association (APTA) will answer questions about back pain over a toll free telephone hot line, 1-800-950-1005, March 6 - 10, 9 a.m. to 5 p.m. Eastern Standard Time (EST).

According to Jane Mathews, president of APTA, the hot line was created to make the public more aware of the importance of back care.

"Over 80 percent of this county's adult population will suffer from back pain some time in their lives, and back pain can greatly effect the quality of an individual's life. The key is often prevention," Mathews said.

According to Jonathan Cooperman, Public Relations Committee Chair for the APTA Section on Orthopedics, for those who already have back problems, the hot line may offer some relief.

"With a physical therapy program, most people with back problems can learn to minimize or eliminate back pain. A lot of our job is educating patients to care for their own backs, but we always recommend that a patient get a professional opinion before starting any kind of exercise or treatment program," he said.

The American Physical Therapy Association is a professional organization serving its 49,000 physical therapist members and the public by fostering improvements in physical therapy education, practice, and research.

-30-

Source: Courtesy of American Physical Therapy Association, Alexandria, Virginia.

peers in the medical community. Unlike advertising and selling, public speaking provides an educational and informative service to the audience, which increases its acceptability. A professional's expertise speaks for itself as he or she delivers a speech.

Meeting an audience face to face before, during, and after a speech personalizes the service and makes the message tangible. Because health care is an intangible service, consumers must rely on other factors to make the decision to use a clinic's service. They rely heavily on word-of-mouth recommendations from friends and relatives, referral from other health care practitioners whom they already trust, and promotional benefits that match what they think they need. A consumer who meets a therapist face to face and listens to the therapist give a speech forms opinions about the care that the therapist provides. Knowledgeability, warmth, and ability to communicate medical facts in lay terms are all transmitted while the therapist speaks and will be remembered when the consumer needs physical therapy.

Another benefit of public speaking is the opportunity for the therapist to select the target audience (Exhibit 4-17). Knowing exactly who will be there, a therapist can target comments to meet the audience members' needs and describe the benefits of physical therapy as they may need it. In addition, the therapist is introduced to this group as an expert so that he or she begins the speech with a marketing edge.

From a marketing perspective, a personal speech reveals a great deal about the therapist, the clinic that he or she represents, and the profession. The audience will draw conclusions about the clinic's image based on the therapist's dress, promotions, style, and speech content. The speech should be designed to educate, inform, or persuade, and its content should promote a positive image.

A speech is often an opportunity to promote the clinic's differential advantages. If it is at all appropriate to include the clinic's differences from its competitors in clinical approaches, experience, location, or equipment, doing so does the audience a service while strengthening the clinic's position in the community.

Overcoming the Fear

Although the thought of speaking before a group is always somewhat frightening, overcoming the fear and giving a well-received speech is exhilarating. (See Exhibit 4-18 for tips on overcoming your fears.) Organizations such as Toastmasters and Dale Carnegie classes provide an opportunity for therapists to learn to speak in a nonthreatening environment. The preparation time required for early

---

Exhibit 4-17 Benefits of Public Speaking

- Creates an accepted, traditional method of practice promotion
- Projects personalized message
- Makes your service tangible
- Allows you to select your target audience
- Introduces you as an expert
- Promotes an image directly and powerfully
- Educates and informs target audiences
- Reinforces your differential advantage and position in the community

Exhibit 4-18 Overcoming the Fear

• Start with small groups	• Start with short speeches
• Start with familiar people	• Practice frequently

speeches may be discouraging, but much of the preparation will become second nature with practice. Just as clinical evaluations take less time with experience, so do speech preparations.

Some therapists start by speaking in front of small groups of people whom they know. For example, a therapist can give an educational in-service presentation to co-workers on a recent seminar. Even in a short speech such as this, the speaker should try to make the message interesting and memorable. A therapist who practices in an institutional setting, such as a hospital or nursing home, can volunteer to give speeches on familiar topics to individuals whom he or she does not know well, to teach patient transfer and positioning techniques to nursing aides, or to participate in new employee orientation.

A therapist can also give speeches to nursing staff on topics of mutual concern. The nursing staff requires monthly in-service programs and may be delighted at such an offer. Physicians also often have monthly educational programming. A physical therapist can begin by teaming up with a well-respected medical staff member for a joint speech. Speeches appropriate for this group include a discussion of clinical research performed in physical therapy or an explanation of high-technology equipment used in physical therapy, such as isokinetic equipment, laser technology, galvanic stimulation, or microvolt stimulation. Well-prepared, informative, and entertaining speeches ensure return invitations to speak to the medical staff again.

Once successful in-house, a therapist is ready to ''take the show on the road'' and speak to groups in the community. If a physical therapy clinic treats rheumatic disease, the Arthritis Foundation has prepared slides and speeches and will arrange speaking appointments for the clinic's therapists. In Washington, D.C., the foundation often places speakers at elder day care and senior centers. Other local and state foundations and associations for diseases and illnesses treated in the clinic may also have prepared materials available. At the very least, they will provide brochures that contain statistics and facts needed to introduce the topic in a speech.

In order to obtain additional speaking practice and to establish themselves as experts in their own professional community, physical therapists may volunteer to speak for their local chapter of the APTA. Topics of interest to fellow professionals include review of anatomy; dysfunctions; and various treatment techniques, combined with successful case studies. The topic may be unique, such as Lyme disease, or common, such as the shoulder, knee, or foot. If a therapist treats a population for whom a new approach to rehabilitation has been developed (e.g., premature infants or those with stroke, cerebral palsy, or head injury), other physical therapists will be interested. Often, that which is routine in one clinic is unique in others. The program coordinator of the local APTA chapter will know which areas of expertise are of interest to the organization.

A therapist who has made several successful, well-received speeches is ready to incorporate public speaking into the marketing plan. A speech is an appropriate marketing tool for a target market any point in the hierarchy of effects. A speech is a good way to introduce a therapist or a clinic. As they give speeches, therapists have a captive audience to whom they can promote their clinic's position and image by their dress, their personality, and their professionalism. Even their punctuality in arriving on time, ending on time, and having time for questions will reinforce the marketing message.

Selection of the Target Audience

One of the first steps in developing a marketing plan is to select the target market(s) (see Chapter 1). Then a therapist can decide when and for what marketing reason in the hierarchy of effects he or she should make a speech. Preparing and giving a speech, not to mention the effort required to obtain an invitation to speak, takes much planning and time (Exhibit 4-19). Therefore, it is essential to be sure that any speaking engagement fits the clinic's marketing plan.

A physical therapist who is ready to use public speaking as a marketing tool should begin by determining when the target market meets as a group and how frequently they invite speakers. For example, if the target market is composed of rheumatologists, the therapist should find out if they have monthly meetings and what type of speakers they invite. If the clinic's specialty is pediatric orthopaedics, the therapist should determine if the Parent-Teachers Association (PTA) in the community welcomes speakers at its meetings. Topics such as scoliosis screening or pediatric sports injuries may interest this group. If your target market meets as a group, getting yourself invited as a speaker is an excellent marketing accomplish-

---

Exhibit 4-19 How To Line Up Speaking Engagements

- Determine target audiences
- Research where and when they meet
- Create a brochure and cover letter
- Contact program organizer/president by phone
- Volunteer for local groups
- List topics that are current and interesting

ment. Your appearance in person and your speech reflect your clinic's image and will position you with your target market as the expert to seek out when your target market has a physical dysfunction you can treat.

Although it is always flattering to be asked to speak, a therapist must be sure that giving a speech fits some aspect of the clinic's marketing plan before accepting the invitation. For example, if the clinic's marketing drive this year is to increase sports physical therapy referrals and a therapist is asked to address a fund raiser for multiple sclerosis, it may be necessary to decline the invitation in spite of its appeal. On the other hand, if the fund raiser for multiple sclerosis is a big media event in the community, making the speech publicizes the honor of the invitation and may reach other target audiences. Furthermore, if the clinic has a neurological division that would benefit from increased visibility, it may be advisable to accept this invitation. If so, however, the speaker or another therapist in the clinic must follow up this speech with a feature in a newsletter, a direct mailing, or follow-up telephone calls. Isolated marketing efforts do not bring a target market through the hierarchy of effects sufficiently to ensure referrals. In accepting the invitation to speak at the fund raiser for multiple sclerosis, the therapist has committed to a marketing campaign to this group. Therefore, it is important to be sure that the clinic and staff have the necessary resources, both financial and energetic, before accepting this invitation to speak. No therapist should make a speech just because the opportunity occurs to do so—unless the therapist needs practice—because it may drain effort, focus, and energy from the clinic's primary target marketing effort.

Most speeches given as publicity for a physical therapy clinic are free. The time involved is an indirect cost of marketing efforts, but the return on investment can be tremendous. Many community groups such as the Kiwanis, the Rotary Club, and even the small business association have small budgets and are delighted to find entertaining and informative free speakers. The following are groups that typically look for speakers and may fit a clinic's marketing plan:

- civic groups, such as Kiwanis and Rotary Club
- large, self-insured employers, such as IBM, MCI, and banks
- national associations, such as the Arthritis Foundation, the American Cancer Society, and the American Heart Association
- health classes, such as those on prenatal care and stress control
- professional and business organizations, such as local chapters of the American Medical Association and unions
- senior centers and retirement communities
- social groups, such as the Parent-Teachers Association
- community organizations, such as sports clubs (e.g., runners' clubs, ski clubs, and hiking clubs)

Speech Preparation

Once an appropriate target audience has been selected, the topic of the speech must be chosen. Topics that may be considered are

- getting in shape
- injury prevention
- the fitness triad: flexibility, strength, endurance
- stress control
- osteoporosis exercises
- arthritis and joint protection
- runner's injuries
- racquet sports shoulder injuries
- caring for the aging parent
- teen fitness
- reducing job-related overuse injuries
- exercise and weight loss

Topics for the Target Market

The target audience determines the appropriate topic and slant of a speech. The therapist should speak to the listeners in their language and from their point of view. If speaking to a group at a diet center about exercise, for example, the therapist should include many references to the contribution of regular exercise to weight loss to make the speech more memorable for this particular group. In a similar lecture on exercise to marathon runners, however, weight loss will be a minor issue; in this case, the therapist should focus on endurance training and injury rehabilitation and prevention.

While outlining a speech, therapists should put themselves in the shoes of the listener in order to learn how to get their points across most effectively and memorably. It is helpful to establish some linkage between a speaker and the audience to demonstrate the speaker's understanding of the issues in the mind of the listeners. Personal anecdotes about fitness training, experiences with an elderly patient, or case examples of patients can help the audience identify with the speaker and listen more closely to the message.

It is often useful to ask the program organizer about audience demographics. Demographic characteristics to consider are age, sex, income, hobbies, sports interests, occupation, and the goals and purposes of the group. This information can sensitize the speech to the special interests and characteristics of the audience.

Type of Speech

A speech can be informative, persuasive, humorous, or a combination. The program coordinator can provide some guidance concerning the group's preference. Unless giving a keynote speech or an awards banquet speech, a physical therapist rarely gives a speech that is primarily humorous. A sprinkle of humor from time to time in even the most serious speech helps to keep the audience's attention from wandering, however.

Informative speeches are most common. They hold no surprises for the audience and provide information in a logical and educational manner. For example, an informative speech is appropriate for members of a jogging club interested in simple ways to prevent injuries. Following standard speech-writing rules, the therapist begins by telling the audience what he or she is going to say and why; continues the body of the speech, repeating the major points periodically to make them memorable; and concludes by again telling the audience what he or she has said (Exhibit 4-20).

In contrast, a persuasive speech appeals to surprise and emotion for the purpose of changing attitudes or behavior. A therapist may give a persuasive speech, for example, to encourage exercise in a sedentary, cardiac disease–prone group. Persuasive speeches begin by establishing credibility through the therapist's credentials (Exhibit 4-21). Human interest case studies are then used to establish the importance of the therapist's point of view. The audience should learn why the

---

Exhibit 4-20 Informative Speech

An informative speech should:

- state what you're going to say
- say it
- conclude by recapping what you said

Exhibit 4-21 Persuasive Speech

A persuasive speech should:

- establish credibility
- tell human interest stories
- appeal to the emotions
- discuss the benefits of changed behavior and/or attitudes
- tell the audience what they can do

topic is important by means of the speech's appeal to their emotions. The therapist should then give suggestions on improving health or preventing illnesses through changed attitudes or behaviors.

Time Limit

Even the most rapt student does not hear every word of a favorite teacher's lectures. Audiences fade out and miss much of a speech. The speaker should try not to take this personally, as it is a normal occurrence. Speakers can improve the audience's attention span by announcing exactly how long they plan to speak, how much meeting time is reserved for questions, and if they plan to stay afterward to answer individual questions. Telling an audience how much time the speech will take allows the audience to set a mental time clock of attention. It is important to end a speech at the promised time; after that time has elapsed, the audience will start thinking about their next activities and how much longer the speech will last, rather than its message. Wrapping up comments on time also demonstrates respect for the audience's schedule.

It is important to practice a speech sufficiently beforehand in order to determine its exact length. The speaker should practice both alone and with another person to get feedback and to get used to an audience. Most speakers talk faster when they are nervous. Consciously slowing down by timing each section of a speech helps this potential timing problem.

On the other side of the time limit, it is wise for a speaker to arrive at least an hour ahead of time in case any last minute problems arise. This time gives the speaker an opportunity to check that audiovisual equipment is in working condition and that he or she can be seen and heard from all seats. Before the audience arrives, the speaker should prepare notes and handouts on the podium and become familiar with the room. These preparations should be complete before the first person arrives (usually about fifteen to twenty minutes early) so that the speaker can mingle and meet the audience prior to taking center stage. This helps to personalize the message. Arriving on time also allows the speaker to start on time, which the hosting group will appreciate.

Visual Aids

A presentation can come alive with the use of visual aids, such as handouts, flip charts, slides, overhead transparencies, and video tapes. Used correctly, visual aids underline a speaker's main points and express the speaker's thoughts visually. It takes practice to become comfortable using visual aids, however. It is better not to use them at all than to use them poorly, because they can make a speaker look disorganized, uninformed, and unsure if introduced at the wrong time. Anyone who has ever been at a speech in which the slides were out of synchronization with the speaker knows how confusing and distracting this can be.

A speaker should prepare to give a speech without the benefit of visual aids. Almost anything can go wrong—from a broken slide projector to missing handouts to a forgotten magic marker for the overhead. Even if something goes wrong, it is the speaker's responsibility to provide a good speech. "The show must go on." Staying calmer than the host and being flexible in emergencies are first-rate qualities in speakers and will lead not only to return invitations, but also to positive word of mouth for the speaker's skills.

Handouts

Unless a speech is a short introductory speech or a humorous speech, handouts will be helpful. Handouts are one of the easiest and least expensive visual aids to produce and use (Exhibit 4-22). If at all possible, the audience should have the handouts before the speech begins. The handouts can be placed on individual chairs, handed out during registration, or passed out as the audience enters the room. Taking time away from the speech to distribute handouts leaves the audience bored for several minutes and detracts from the effectiveness of the speech.

A handout should include the title of the speech, the speaker's name, brief background, address, telephone number, and date. It should contain the goals for the speech, as well as the outline and key points. There should be enough space in the outline for the audience to add pertinent notes and comments for future reference. Organized handouts that allow the audience to follow along as the speech is given helps them to understand the message; they listen to the words rather than writing

---

Exhibit 4-22 Handouts

Benefits

- Audience can listen rather than write
- Organizes your speech for the audience
- Tangible reminder of your speech
- Allows greater audience participation

Format

- Outline
- Key points
- Audience participation activity
- Space for notes

Cover Page

- Speech title
- Your name
- Brief background
- Address
- Phone number
- Date

them down. Also, when their attention wanders, as it inevitably will, handouts make it easier for them to find their place in the speech. Handouts provide a tangible souvenir of the speech with the important points highlighted.

Handouts can be sprinkled with audience participation activities. Asking the audience to take a few minutes to complete a questionnaire or brainstorm ideas with a neighbor and write down the results to share with the group engages their participation and increases audience attention span. Giving tasks like this in handouts also helps to personalize the message. Placing activities such as this at 20- or 30-minute intervals keeps the speech interesting and meaningful.

The speaker should be familiar enough with the handouts to refer to points made in the handout during the speech. This increases audience perception of the speaker's organization. Many speakers like to speak directly from the handout. If the speaker prefers to use a more complete text, it may be helpful to make a notation in the margin of the speech at each point where the audience's attention should be drawn to the handout.

If appropriate to the target market, a therapist can include the practice, clinic, or institution brochure for future audience reference, for background information, and for increased name recognition associated with the speech. Depending on the topic, many foundations and nonprofit organizations will provide informational brochures, pamphlets, or fliers for distribution to the audience. These publications are often free. For example, the Arthritis Foundation has free brochures available on many topics from osteoarthritis to lupus erythematosus. The audience will appreciate the speaker's thoughtfulness and effort on their behalf.

Flip Charts

For groups of thirty or fewer, a flip chart can be an excellent visual aid. With larger groups, a flip chart loses its effectiveness because some of the audience cannot see it. Flip charts can be made in advance or written on during the speech. For example, it is often effective to write outline headings, with one or two key points, on the top of the page. Then, during the speech, the speaker can underline key words or write new ones on the page.

A major advantage of flip charts is that they are inexpensive and easy to prepare ahead of time. Furthermore, a flip chart is easily changed to accommodate any changes in the speech. A thick magic marker on a flip chart brings attention to the speaker and his or her comments during the speech. Writing down the audience's comments as they are made encourages audience participation and feedback. One of the primary benefits of using a flip chart is that the lights can stay on, which is beneficial after lunch or late in the afternoon when people tend to be drowsy. Flip charts can also be an excellent change of pace from slides or other visual aids (Exhibit 4-23). A speaker can use a flip chart in the middle of a speech for the purpose of turning on the lights for a while, writing down audience comments, and keeping interest high.

Exhibit 4-23 Flip Charts

Advantages	*Disadvantages*
• Are inexpensive	• May look cheap
• Are easy to prepare ahead	• Can look awkward if not used with ease
• Can be shown with lights on	• Can't travel by airplane
• Enable speaker to write while speaking	
• Are good adjuncts for audience participation	

The primary disadvantage of flip charts that require preparation ahead of time is that they are too large to carry comfortably on airplanes; for speeches given locally, however, they are fine. A speaker must practice sufficiently ahead of time to become comfortable with the medium; otherwise, the speaker may appear awkward when turning slightly away from the audience to write. Because audiences know that flip charts are inexpensive, a therapist's speech presentation and professional persona must be polished.

Overhead Transparencies

Projected on a slide screen in front of the audience, overhead transparencies are inexpensive and can be made from a typed or handwritten page by a camera or slide shop, usually within twenty-four hours. Alternatively, an in-house copier may have the capacity to make them. Overhead transparencies look professional and are easily carried in a briefcase or notebook. Because a speaker can write on a transparency during a speech, it makes a good adjunct to audience participation. (See Exhibit 4-24 for advantages and disadvantages in using transparencies.)

Exhibit 4-24 Overhead Transparencies

Advantages	*Disadvantages*
• Are inexpensive	• Audience lights must be dim
• Are professional looking	• Require a microphone and stage with a clear path from the podium to the projector
• Are lightweight and easy to carry in a briefcase	
• Enable speaker to write while speaking	
• Are good adjuncts for audience participation	
• Can be projected on a screen for large audiences	

The use of transparencies for an entire presentation, if it is longer than fifteen to twenty minutes, can feel repetitious and boring to the audience. It is better to turn the overhead off and bring the lights up from time to time during the speech, just to vary the presentation style and add interest.

A therapist who wants to use overhead transparencies during a speech should check the facility with a member of the host group first. The microphone must have a cord sufficiently long to stretch from the podium to the projector, and the path from the podium to the projector must be clear and must not require the speaker to jump up and down off a stage. Otherwise, the speaker may appear awkward while moving about to use the equipment and may be invisible to the audience if it is necessary to speak while standing off the stage.

As with the use of other visual aids, it is essential to practice using transparencies. It is also helpful to practice switching from the use of the overhead projector to other phases of the speech to ensure smooth, professional transitions.

Slides

Accompanying a speech with slides enhances the presentation and adds professional polish. There are many ways to use slides. Word slides can be mixed with picture slides for a varied presentation. Some speakers like to use two slide projectors, showing words on one screen and pictures on another.

To become comfortable using slides while they speak, some therapists volunteer to speak for an organization that has a prepared script and slide presentation. Local organizations such as The Arthritis Foundation or the YMCA, for example, may have prepared presentations that can be used for initial practice. Large institutions sometimes have public or in-house presentations prepared to be given by staff, and those who work for these institutions may be able to use these presentations.

Producing slides for a presentation can be costly. The least expensive method is for speakers to take their own. If a therapist's presentation is clinical in nature, he or she may take many slides of patients, clinic, and staff. In order to use pictures of patients, however, it is necessary to get signed release forms; these forms should be kept on file with the script (Exhibit 4-25).

A camera with a macrolens and small tripod can be used to take slides of typed pages or professionally produced graphics. In the latter case, the source must be credited on the slide. Word slides should each contain only a few words or a short sentence, as a slide filled with words is difficult for audiences to read and detracts from the presentation. Word slides taken in this manner look like a typed page, black print on white background. For approximately $4.00 per slide, typed pages can be professionally made into slides with white printing on blue background. This process is called "blue foil." In this method, the words are enlarged to fit the slide so that they are easier to read from a distance.

Exhibit 4-25 Photograph Release Form

I understand that the pictures taken today may be used in educational speeches. I consent to
this.

_____   _____
Witness   Patient

                                          _____
                                          Date

Professional graphics design and four-color slides look the best. They generally cost between $15 and $30 each, but can cost as much as $300 depending on the experience, skill, and demand of the graphic designer. A therapist who plans to repeat a speech several times may want to have a title and conclusion slide made at first and add one or two slides of this type each time. If the speech is to be made before a prestigious group or will be repeated often, it may be worthwhile to have the slides professionally prepared.

Before preparing the slides, the speaker should write and practice the speech several times. Slides should be changed every thirty seconds to two minutes, which means that there should be a slide for every four or five lines of written text. Varying the length of time that slides are on the screen helps maintain audience interest. Occasionally, a slide may remain on the screen longer than two minutes or less than thirty seconds for variety.

The placement of the slides should be noted in the text of the speech. The number and content of each slide can be written in the margin for easy placement in the slide carousel. This notation is also extremely helpful if the speaker loses his or her place in the speech, or if the slides are out of order for some reason. Referring to the notations in the margin allows the speaker to get back on track with minimal interruption of the speech.

The speaker should underline or highlight in a bright color the word on which the slide is to be changed. It is very distracting when the slide does not match the text of the speech. The audience is thinking more about why the slide has not changed when the speaker has moved to another topic or when the speaker will move to the new information presented by the slide. Timing slides with a speech becomes very easy and almost subconscious with practice.

Videotape

It is inadvisable to use videotape for an entire presentation, because it depersonalizes the message and removes the all-important audience-speaker dynamic relationship. Videotape shown through a television monitor can effectively bring a physical therapy clinic to the audience, however. VHS is the format most commonly available in hotels and convention centers.

Videotape can illustrate patient evaluation or treatment techniques, exercise or stretching routines, home programs, or patient education. It can be produced by the clinic's staff with a rented camera if the clinic does not own a camera. All that is needed is a steady hand and the ability to edit unnecessary footage. A homemade videotape is a perfectly acceptable way to illustrate a point made in the speech. These illustrations should be short, however. The attention span of television viewers is twenty seconds for commercials and five minutes for programming. "Home movies" can be boring, but a short clip can increase audience interest, diversion, and emphasize a point quite well.

A twenty-minute videotape produced professionally, when the clinic staff provides the basic script, can take a day to a week to shoot and can cost approximately $1,000 per finished minute. Depending on the importance of the speech and the frequency with which therapists plan to use the videotape, this cost may be justifiable.

The Performance

Professional Image

The way in which speakers project themselves, from the moment that they are greeted by the first person to the moment that they shake hands with the last person, influences the image that they leave behind. Projection includes clothes and how well they fit, hair and how it is styled, manner and how they carry themselves. Image is even influenced by attitude, posture, and speaking accent (Exhibit 4-26). Not only do clothes need to fit well and be styled to match audience expectation, but also the speaker should look comfortable and at ease in them.

If planning to wear a new outfit, the speaker should practice the speech wearing it until he or she feels comfortable. New shoes should be broken in until the speaker can stand without noticing them for the length of their speech; uncomfort-

---

Exhibit 4-26 Professional Image

A professional image includes:

- Clothes
- Hairstyle
- Manner

- Attitude
- Posture
- Accent

able shoes are distracting. If planning to change hairstyles, the new one should be tried out several months ahead so that it can be changed if unsatisfactory. Hair should be cut about two weeks before the speech to avoid that newly cut, too short look.

Projecting a positive, good-natured attitude personalizes the speaker and helps the audience feel comfortable. Even posture and carriage speak nonverbally to the audience. An erect posture, with the center of gravity directly over the feet and a strong, grounded stance, projects a self-assured image. It may help to imagine professional speakers who have been impressive and try to incorporate their attributes into a speaking performance.

Use of Notes

Speeches can be memorized, typed or written in outline form, highlighted on note cards, or typed out verbatim. The best style of notes is the most comfortable style for the speaker. Memorizing a speech with the use of notes for reference allows the speaker more freedom to communicate with the audience through eye contact and gestures; the speaker can move from behind the podium and be more expressive. The speaker who has memorized a speech, however, has no crutch if a point is forgotten or the place in the speech is lost. A speech should be memorized only when the speaker has a photographic memory, the speech is short, or the speaker is very experienced.

The outline is a good format from which to speak for several reasons. Speakers cannot bury their noses in the text when it is in outline form. They must be familiar enough with the subject to be able to speak somewhat extemporaneously, given key thoughts from the outline. Because extemporaneous speaking usually has more voice inflection and change of pace than reading directly from a text, it increases audience interest and participation in the subject.

Many speakers like to use note cards, as they are easy to handle and read. It is common for a speaker to put one or two thoughts on each note card and speak extemporaneously from those thoughts. Details can be written on the back of the card in case the speaker loses the train of thought or forgets a point. A brief pause while the speaker refers to the back of the note card is seldom noticed by the audience. The note cards should be numbered in case they fall or become mixed in sequence.

Some speakers like to use completely typed speeches with key thoughts high-lighted in order to keep them on track. This approach is particularly beneficial for the beginning speaker, who can refer to the entire text during brief periods of stage fright. Speeches given to people who speak another language and require simul-taneous translation must be typed verbatim. The speech is given to the translators ahead of time, with notations for slide positions so that exact meaning can be maintained.

Setting the Tone

A speech should begin with an icebreaker, such as a short story or joke, that helps to connect the speaker with the audience and captures the audience's attention. The speaker should have a prepared icebreaker, but should be ready to change it if a better story comes along that morning. Anything that is similar between the audience and the speaker is appropriate. For example, "I was born in this town, and what I remember best about it is . . . ." or "My father was a Mason, and he always said. . . ." The similar connection icebreaker should be a current experience, such as "In the car on the way over. . . ." If the speaker is a good joke teller, a joke can be an excellent way to start a speech. The icebreaker should last no more than two to three minutes.

After the icebreaker, the speaker should review the speech's objectives with the audience, give the outline, and announce break times and exhibit times. In this way, the audience has a chance to modify their expectations for the speech initially rather than waiting until the end to hear something that is not going to be presented. The speaker should clearly indicate how and when questions will be answered, including whether individual questions will be answered after the speech.

From the start, the speaker must establish and maintain rapport with the audience. Eye contact and a few gestures are helpful. Looking at one or two people while speaking is more comfortable than speaking to a sea of faces, and the audience will perceive that the speaker is personalizing the message for them. The speaker should smile, relax, and talk *to* the audience, not *at* them. Talking down to an audience will cause them to "tune out." During the speech, it is helpful occasionally to monitor the facial and body language reactions of the audience.

It can be difficult for a speaker to keep the attention of an audience used to the polished presentations of electronic media. Depending on audience reaction, the speaker can vary the pacing by speaking fast, then slowly; loudly then softly. A good way to keep the audience's attention is to make a few points, then tell a story to illustrate the point. For example, in a speech to elders at a day care center about life style modification in arthritis, the speaker can illustrate the point by telling a story about a patient who continued to have pain until she spread out her chores with rest periods and varying activities. Stories can make points come alive.

Speakers, being human, make mistakes. If handled with humor, mistakes can actually foster good will with the audience. A sincere and friendly attitude is more important than perfection. Speakers should let the audience laugh with them at their mistakes.

The speech should conclude with a restatement of the goals and a summary of the main points. The floor may be opened for questions if time is available. The speaker should then thank the audience and the host. See Exhibit 4-27 for a summary of speaking tips.

A physical therapist should follow up a speech with a letter to obtain feedback on the performance and also to remind the audience of the clinic's service. Speaker

Exhibit 4-27 Speaking Tips

- Begin with an icebreaker
- Establish a connection between yourself and the audience
- State your goals and expectations
- Involve your audience
- Establish time limit and breaks
- State how and when questions will be entertained
- Smile, relax, and talk to the audience, not at them
- Be sincere and friendly. This is more important than being perfect. Let them laugh with you at your mistakes.
- Vary presentation style to maintain audience attention using voice inflection, speed, and volume
- Make points, then tell stories
- Use A-Vs to make points and capture attention
- Conclude by stating goals and summarizing main points
- Practice

surveys are commonly distributed by the host (Exhibit 4-28). Depending on the size and nature of the audience, a therapist can follow up with telephone calls or letters to participants as appropriate.

Example of a Speech

The following speech was prepared for the participants of a media relations workshop held in June of 1988 by the Private Practice Section of the American Physical Therapy Association.*

Slowing the Spiral: The Physical Therapist's Role in Curbing Health Care Costs

It's hard to pick up a business publication these days without seeing a reference to the increasing cost of health-care. And national studies predict that the price tag for companies to provide health-care coverage for employees will continue to rise. In response, many companies are developing new strategies to deal with these expanding costs.

More and more, companies are turning to the physical therapist for professional guidance in this area. This reliance has grown markedly

Source: Developed by Brouillard Communications for the Private Practice Section of the American Physical Therapy Association, 1988. Reprinted with permission.

Exhibit 4-28 Speaker Evaluation Form

---

1. Rate the overall presentation:
   _____ Excellent   _____ Good   _____ Fair   _____ Poor
   Comments:_____

2. The speaker's topic was
   _____ Stimulating   _____ Interesting
   _____ Slightly interesting   _____ Boring
   Comments:_____

3. The speaker's presentation skill was
   _____ Excellent   _____ Good   _____ Fair   _____ Poor
   Comments: _____

4. Content covered was
   _____ Too complex   _____ Just right   _____ Too simple
   Comments: _____

5. Use of audiovisual aids was
   _____ Excellent   _____ Good   _____ Fair   _____ Poor
   Comments: _____

6. I would like to hear this speaker again.
   _____ Yes   _____ No
   Comments: _____

7. Other topics of interest to me:
   _____
   _____
   _____

---

over the last decade as the physical therapist's traditional function as a health care provider has evolved.

During this period of professional expansion, physical therapists across the country have introduced programs that extend well beyond their basic role of designing and carrying out rehabilitation programs. The new emphasis is on preventing injuries in the first place and avoiding the re-injury of returning workers.

These are important areas of attention because worker-injury costs are a large part of industrial America's health-care bill. In 1980, the U.S. government reported that all worker compensation benefits paid in that year totalled over 13 billion dollars. By 1984, the figure had grown to nearly 20 billion. And by 1985, it was 22½ billion dollars. That upward cost trend is continuing today.

How do workers get injured? There are three common causes—lifting, repetitive motions and vibrations. The result in each case is pain and suffering that results from what the physical therapist calls a "musculoskeletal" disorder.

Injuries to the lower back are the most common, and most of these are caused by lifting or other load handling. They account for 20% of all occupational injuries and one-third of all compensation costs. In other words, each year 1 out of 50 American industrial workers suffers a lower-back injury.

Lower-back injuries are usually caused by lifting or other load handling. While these injuries are usually quite painful, most are fortunately not permanent. In fact, four out of five workers return to the job in three weeks. Nonetheless, estimates place the total loss from these disorders and their related expenses at more than 14 billion dollars a year.

While lower-back injuries dominate the roster of workplace mishaps, other disorders also are producing significant suffering and cost. Two major ones, tendonitis and "carpal tunnel syndrome," have been traced to patterns of repetitive motions and vibrations.

Tendonitis results from tears in the tendon that become inflamed and painful. "Tennis elbow" is a familiar example of tendonitis in the sports world, but the disorder can afflict almost any tendon that is heavily stressed.

Carpal tunnel syndrome is a less familiar injury that disables the hand. Named for a narrow tunnel in the wrist formed by ligaments and bone, carpal tunnel syndrome is caused by the repetition of stressful hand motions. The carpal tunnel houses the median nerve and tendons that close the hand. When a worker performs repeated stressful hand motions, the tendons swell and apply pressure to the median nerve. If this condition goes untreated, it leads to muscle deterioration, loss of grip and crippling of the hand. Advanced cases can be irreversible.

For all of these disorders, the physical therapist advocates preventive measures and a complete program of injury management. The savings produced by these two programs far outweigh their cost to employers. That's hardly surprising when you consider that the average cost per back injury, for example, is 6,000 dollars.

Indeed, the savings derived from the use of physical therapy have been graphically illustrated in a number of cases found in a recent study that the Washington Business Group on Health conducted for the Private Practice Section of the American Physical Therapy Association.

For example, the Adolph Coors Company reports savings of over 600,000 dollars as a result of programs for the treatment of back and orthopedic conditions among its employees.

General Motors Corporation has documented savings of 354 work weeks plus 25,000 dollars in associated costs during the first year GM provided a rehabilitation, work hardening and health awareness program to its Detroit-area employees. And the Potomac Electric Power Company estimates that its orthopedic program saves the utility approximately 500,000 dollars each year.

An ideal preventive program starts with the worker—and it would begin even before employment with a screening by a designated member of the personnel department. To do that screening, the personnel interviewer uses an assessment tool that physical therapists have recently developed. It's called the functional job description. It spells out a job's physical demands and specifically its musculoskeletal requirements. The best descriptions will also include a videotape of the job being performed.

To match their jobs to candidates, employers examine candidates against three performance criteria—range-of-motion, strength and endurance. Long-term studies are now under way to firmly establish the validity of each of these standards.

Despite what statistics may suggest, injuries are not inevitable. Many can be reduced or eliminated. And a good place to start is where people do the work. The workplace and the tasks that are performed in it can be designed to fit the worker. Whether this concept is called human engineering or ergonomics, the aim is the same—to minimize injuries that result from workplace activities.

In some cases, changing the workplace is not feasible. When this is true, physical therapists turn to other strategies to reduce injuries. Take training, for example. When workers are educated about body mechanics and safe work habits, they become alert to hazards. The net effect is usually a reduction in the scale and scope of injuries. Some physical therapists are extending the effectiveness of training by developing specialized courses for specific occupations. For example, they teach transfer training to nurses, lifting procedures to stock handlers and posture to deskbound office workers.

America's emphasis on physical fitness is helping workers, too. This relatively new awareness of the importance of health maintenance techniques has prepared employers to accept the value of fitness in reducing injuries. Many companies now pay all or part of employee memberships in gyms and fitness programs. Again, physical therapists are extending the benefits of these workout programs by creating specialized sets of exercises to meet the work tolerance levels of particular jobs.

Physical therapists have also introduced the idea of exercise breaks in the workplace itself. These brief but regular sessions include exercises of the body parts that undergo special stress on the job. We have early indications that such sessions can do a lot to reduce the muscle trauma commonly caused by repetitive tasks.

While all of these preventive measures are helping to reduce injuries, hundreds of thousands of workers are still temporarily disabled each year. For these traditional clients, the physical therapist designs rehabilitation programs and personally helps the injured workers follow these regimens.

Today, these standard rehabilitation programs still make up the bulk of the profession's work. However, the increasing cost of downtime has made the physical therapist sensitive to the need for techniques that will return employees to their jobs and keep them there—without in any way increasing risk to them.

The jobs that injured workers return to can enhance or inhibit their recovery. So those tasks must be chosen carefully. The wrong work can re-injure workers, and the chronic disorders that can result can become lifelong trials to the workers and built-in costs for employers. Back injuries are the classic example. About 20% of persistent back pains account for 80% of the dollars spent on all back disorders.

One of the tools the physical therapist is using to assess a returning worker's job-readiness is the Functional Capacities Evaluation (FCE). Basically, it is a comprehensive test of a person's ability to perform specific work without adverse reaction. Conversely, the test also notes those tasks the worker *cannot* perform with ease. The FCE is a comparatively new technique, yet it has already positively affected the return-to-work process for many workers.

While an FCE tests total physical functioning, it always includes the full range of tasks the worker must deal with on the job. The test itself takes several hours, during which the therapist stresses the worker's physical capacities to the maximum. The results of an FCE provide a measurable level of safe job activity that forecasts the worker's productivity and indicates tasks that must be modified or eliminated to prevent re-injury.

There is another benefit of a Functional Capacities Evaluation. It indicates whether a returning employee must physically prepare, or train, as it were, to resume work.

If such "work-hardening" preparation is required, the physical therapist creates a custom-tailored regimen. It will include the specific tasks that were part of the FCE test.

Because an FCE shows workers what they can and cannot do, they can better understand the extent of their recovery and how they can avoid re-injury. This information puts them in control and does a great deal to dispel inhibiting fears. As a result, most workers take a more active part in the effort to return them to normal activity.

The cost of health care is the driving force behind innovation in the worker-injury area. Many employers have excellent programs, such as those to curb back injuries and re-evaluate work stations. The physical therapist is a member of the team that's making these very welcome improvements. At the same time, these traditional health care providers are creating the next wave of innovations that employers need to slow the health-cost spiral.

MEDIA INTERVIEWS

Many people shudder at the very thought of speaking in public. In fact, the fear of public speaking comes before the fear of death and the fear of taxes in the heart of the average person. Most fears of public speaking and interviews can be overcome by practice and by the self-confidence that comes from knowing more on the subject than the audience or interviewer, however. Therefore, an invitation to be interviewed by the media should be accepted as a challenge.

Benefits of Media Interviews

Physical therapy needs professionals to speak with the media to publicize physical therapy and to bring the profession once and for all out of the basement and into the community. The average U.S. citizen does not know what physical therapists do, what the benefits of their services are, or how to gain access to their services. Therefore, many citizens are suffering unnecessarily with functional restrictions, pain, stiffness, scar tissue adhesions, and movement disorders. Many people could be treated and healed if they knew about physical therapy.

As more physical therapists are interviewed on television and radio or in newspapers and magazines, the public will better understand the benefits of therapy. With improved understanding will come more appropriate referrals, earlier interventions, increased patient satisfaction, and greater public visibility of physical therapy. Each physical therapist who accepts the professional challenge to overcome interview anxiety and speak out to the media benefits not only the professional image, but also the members of the public who are unaware of how they can benefit from physical therapy.

Definition of a Good Interview

The basis of every good interview is the projection of a positive attitude. The therapist's words, phrases, and facial expressions should all express this attitude toward the subject, profession, and life. The therapist should make it clear to the interviewer that he or she is happy to be involved in the interview, cares about physical therapy, and is an authority on the subject. In addition, the therapist should try to speak in short punchy sentences that are quotable. Thinking and speaking as if writing a headline rather than discussing a topic in detail will keep the listeners interested. We are a society that communicates rapidly; we are used to short, thirty- and even 15-second spot commercials.

Some of the terms that physical therapists use every day are incomprehensible to the general public. Therefore, a physical therapist who is being interviewed should avoid using jargon that is not familiar to most people. The term *thigh* can replace the term *femur*; the term *treatment technique* can replace the term *modality*. Although it is important to have an air of authority, the audience will not listen if they do not understand the terminology.

Good News

Therapists should consider media interviewers as the target market when determining newsworthy items and should mentally place themselves in the position of a reporter who is competing for the public interest with other forms of media, as well as with competitors in the same medium. Because the news media are businesses with a bottom line of profitability and ratings, the purpose of news stories related to health issues is to advise, inform, and entertain. Of critical importance to the viewers (listeners/readers) is that the news is understandable from the point of view of their own concerns. Therefore, the reporter's target market is the news consumer. When attempting to gain visibility through interviews, a physical therapist should discuss the topic with the reporter in terms of consumer interest, competitor news items, informational content, entertainment value, and the power of the story to draw an audience.

There are five basic areas of news in reporting, and each can be applied to physical therapy.

1. new technology
2. new way to solve an old problem
3. human interest
4. controversy
5. current events

A new electrical pain control device or isokinetic exercise equipment may be newsworthy new technology. A new type of brace that is more lightweight or easier to mold for use in rehabilitation than are the older types may be of interest to the general public as a new way to solve an old problem, particularly if a newsworthy person has a condition that could use this brace. For example, if a well-known football player suffers a knee injury on the field, he may benefit from this new brace.

Every newspaper, television news program, and radio show has a human interest section. Human interest stories may involve case studies and success stories, such as the relief of someone's chronic pain through physical therapy. It may be helpful to obtain a testimonial from that person. If that person is familiar to the public, the item will be all the more newsworthy.

News consumers often identify with an underdog and enjoy watching a reporter stand up for the underdog's cause. Although therapists should in general be careful not to portray themselves as pitiable, it may at times be appropriate to do so. For example, an individual practitioner or a therapist in a small private practice who is being interviewed may discuss the increasing difficulties in getting referrals, while the health care giants, such as hospitals, health maintenance organizations, and physician groups, capture the market.

Controversy is always newsworthy. Because it may shed a positive or negative light, however, it may be wise to avoid controversy. For example, a therapist may not want to talk about the controversy between therapists and chiropractors. First of all, physical therapists are not qualified to talk about what chiropractors do or do not do; they are qualified only to talk about their own specialty. Second, any controversy between physical therapists and chiropractors is not likely to be a major item on a therapist's agenda, and discussing the issue may waste precious interview time. In order to stay away from newsworthy topics that they do not wish to discuss, therapists should have several newsworthy ideas of their own.

Listening to the morning news and reading at least two newspapers prior to the interview may reveal events related to an item to be discussed during the interview. The therapist should plan to bring the interview around to that particular current event and its relationship to physical therapy.

Preparation for an Interview

In recognizing and knowing what the media consider news, the therapist has taken the first step in preparing for the interview. It is also important to know the style of reporting preferred by the reporter as well as the preferred topics and items he or she has covered in the past. To prepare formally, the therapist should write down a personal agenda and the items that he or she wants to get across in the interview. It may be necessary to turn the interviewer's questions around to this agenda by using a connecting thought as a bridge. For example, a pediatric physical therapist who wishes to discuss the need for public funding support of rehabilitation at an early age may respond to an interviewer's question about football injuries by saying,

> "Rehabilitation of football injuries has made tremendous advances in recent years. In the past, prior to good protective equipment, such as padded helmets, football players were prone to head injuries which sometimes caused them to lose control over their bodies, much as children who are born with developmental disabilities are unable to control their limbs. Did you know that there is a severe problem in this community with lack of funding for rehabilitation of children with developmental disabilities?"

Almost every question can in some way be turned around to meet the therapist's agenda. It is important not to ignore any question, but to answer it briefly and then try to bridge onto an agenda topic. Sending the interviewer a list of questions that relate to the agenda prior to the interview will help the interviewer prepare for the interview and enhance the therapist's professional image. Exhibit 4-29 includes factors necessary for interview preparation.

Getting an Interview

The first step in getting an interview is to research the local media. It is important to determine whether the target market listens to the radio, watches television, reads the newspaper, or subscribes to magazines in order to obtain health news. It is also important to determine what time of day the members of this group most frequently use the media. For example, those over the age of sixty-five generally watch the early evening news on television and are more likely to watch television after midnight than are their younger, employed counterparts. If this age

---

Exhibit 4-29 Interview Preparation

- Project a professional image
- Know your audience
- Know your reporter
- List your own agenda
- Send interviewer preparatory questions
- Research current events that relate to your agenda

group is the target market, the therapist should research various competitive media options with those time frames to determine which one(s) are preferable for an interview.

Once the therapist has targeted the appropriate media, the next step is to determine who makes the programming or interview decisions. In radio and television, the assignment editor or the news editor makes these decisions. Sometimes it is possible to find out how the editor chooses interviews simply by calling the assignment editor and asking for this information. It may be difficult to reach news editors by telephone, however. These people are under pressure from constant deadlines and numerous special interest groups.

Even if unable to obtain information by telephone, the therapist should do some homework by monitoring the targeted news media for items similar to those on the therapist's agenda. Listening to a local radio station that has a regular health spot, for example, will indicate the type of news that the station is most likely to cover. The station may have a bias toward human interest, prevention, health research, or medical malpractice issues. With this knowledge, the therapist can decide the best approach to take with that particular station.

An introductory letter is appropriate at this point. It should have a descriptive one-line heading that captures the essence of the topic of the potential interview. The body of the letter should contain a concise explanation of who, what, where, when, why, and how an interview will be of interest to the media's constituency. The letter should list the contact person with day and evening telephone numbers.

Within a few days after the letter has arrived, the therapist should follow up with a telephone call to establish the level of interest in the topic. In such telehone calls, therapists should present themselves as friendly, helpful experts. Perhaps if the topic is not of interest at this time, another time or topic will be. Even if the interview idea is rejected, it is important to sound positive and helpful. The reporter may remember the therapist the next time an expert resource is needed for a health story.

Difficult Questions

If an interview turns into an interrogation such as those on ''60 Minutes,'' therapists can handle difficult questions with a three-phase approach.

1. answering the question directly
2. answering the question briefly
3. creating a transition to their own points

If a reporter asks, for example, ''Don't most people believe that chiropractors are the best practitioner for back problems?''

1. direct answer: "Yes, that is a fallacy believed by much of the public."
2. brief answer: "A study published in the *New York Times* found physical therapists to be second only to physiatrists in obtaining long-term positive results in helping people with chronic back pain."
3. transition: "Physical therapists believe that our emphasis on exercise and prevention allows consumers to put health care back in their own hands, where it belongs."

In other words, the therapist should not avoid the question, should not ignore the question, but should turn the topic away from the question as quickly as possible.

There are various techniques that an interviewer may use to throw the person being interviewed off balance. Some reporters ask two or three questions in a row without allowing time for an answer. If a reporter uses this technique, the therapist has no responsibility to remember and answer all the questions in order. All the therapist should do is pick the one question that is closest to an item on his or her agenda and answer it. Some reporters pause, leaving an empty space after the person being interviewed has finished answering the question in the hope that the person will say something untoward. Mike Wallace is famous for using this technique, and it works. During an interview, three seconds feels like five minutes. If the person being interviewed has answered the question, however, it is the interviewer's responsibility to fill the space.

If a therapist is truly caught off guard by an interviewer's question and cannot think of a good way to bridge the question into his or her own agenda, the therapist should say that he or she cannot talk about that issue now, but will meet with the interviewer later to discuss it in detail. It is important never to lie or fudge during an interview; the reporter will realize it and will probe further to determine what the therapist is trying to hide or does not know. It does not hurt to acknowledge an inability to answer a particular question. Honesty is better than any attempt to mislead the interviewer. It is also important to remember that nothing is ever off the record, either before or after the interview. Everything that the therapist says is fair game and may make it into print.

A therapist being interviewed should occasionally make the reporter look good by making remarks such as "That's a very good question" or "I'm glad you asked that." Therapists should always prepare a twenty-second wrap-up of their agenda to use at the end of an interview. It should be interesting, clear, and memorable. It is the final impression that will remain with the audience.

Television Interview Tips

Although it may be difficult to obtain a television interview, the beneficial exposure can be worth the effort. Most people get their news information from television. They consider information imparted through television interviews true and important, as they believe that the reporter must have researched the topic. Because television coverage delivers a message to a large number of people simultaneously, it is a powerful marketing tool.

Television audiences have a thirty-second attention span, so it is necessary to speak in punchy headlines in order to attract and hold the audience's attention. Lengthy and detailed explanations should be avoided unless they are broken up with humor or interesting stories. During a television interview, leaning slightly forward, toward the interviewer, when answering a question conveys confidence and authority. A person being interviewed should always look into the host's eyes, even if the camera may be on someone else. It takes practice and experience to remain professional and calm while looking into the television camera lens. Looking away from the host's eyes or into the viewing monitor on the floor makes a person being interviewed appear to lack self-confidence, and the audience will wonder why that person is looking down at the floor. The head should be kept level in listening and answering questions; tilting the head to the right or left when answering a question is a request for approval in nonverbal language. Arm gestures should be small and below the face, and body language should be open rather than closed. No matter how nervous, the person being interviewed should try not to grab the chair arms, jiggle the legs or fingers, or exhibit any other signs of anxiety.

Colors that work best on television are tans and blues. Very light or very dark colors, stripes, and loud patterns should be avoided. If a microphone is to be worn, women should wear a suit rather than a silk blouse so that the microphone can be pinned to the lapel; a microphone is distracting when pinned on a blouse. No medical jargon should be used. The person being interviewed should maintain concentration at all times, even if the host is speaking to someone else. Finally, if at all possible, an opportunity should be found to use the prepared twenty-second wrap-up at the end of the interview. Television interview tips are listed in Exhibit 4-30.

Radio Interview Tips

Physical therapists should prepare for radio interviews much as they prepare for television interviews: determining the listening audience ahead of time, sending targeted questions ahead to the interviewer, and finding out what interests the reporter and why they were asked to speak on the show. In interviewing on the radio, whether it is a live or taped interview, a therapist should try to pretend that the microphone is not there and speak to the reporter as if he or she were a friend or a patient. This approach helps a person being interviewed to relax and forget that hundreds of nameless, faceless people are listening.

Exhibit 4-30 Television Interview Tips

- Speak in concise sentences
- Lean slightly toward interviewer when speaking
- Look interviewer in eyes
- Wear clothing that accommodates a microphone
- Avoid tilting your head
- Avoid large arm gestures
- Avoid showing nervous habits
- Avoid very light or very dark colors
- Avoid jargon
- Close by summarizing your points briefly

Newspaper Interview Tips

The ultimate goal of media relations with newspaper reporters is to become a regular professional resource, the person whom the reporters call for professional information whenever they have a question concerning physical therapy. The reporters should be told that they need not quote the therapist personally every time that they use him or her as a resource. It is wise for a therapist to send in article ideas frequently, even without being asked, to keep his or her name and expertise in front of the reporters' consciousness constantly.

Ninety percent of newspaper interviews are conducted by telephone. When called by a newspaper reporter for a telephone interview, a therapist is not obligated to speak to that reporter at that time if it is inconvenient. The therapist has the right and obligation to ask the reporter to call back at another time, preferably the same day. When the reporter calls back, the therapist should have other calls and messages held during the interview. In order to remind themselves of the importance of the interview, many therapists stand up during the telephone interview. They may also offer to take the reporter out to lunch so that they can get to know the reporter's needs and interests and will be able to do better follow-up.

CONCLUSION

Physical therapists need to overcome their fear of the media and take the risks necessary to project a positive message and image to the public. Those who plan to do television interviews should rent or borrow a video camera to practice; those who plan to do radio or telephone interviews should use an audiocassette recorder. It is essential to try it, practice it, and master it to spread the word about physical therapy through media interviews.

The public relations efforts described in this chapter are not marketing ends in and of themselves, but are simply marketing tools that can be used in combination to accomplish the marketing goals outlined in the marketing strategic plan. Although many organizations confuse these tools with marketing, the tools do not stand by themselves to promote a physical therapy clinic. A brochure, newsletter, or speech by itself—without a marketing strategy coordinated externally in the community and internally with employees—will rarely have a significant impact on organizational goals. When public relations activities are combined with effective quality service, with professional employees, and, possibly, with selling and advertising, the marketing program will be successful.

NOTES

1. R.S. MacStravic, "Professional and Personal Quality of Care in Health Care Delivery," *Health Marketing Quarterly* 5 (1987/88):125.

2. J.P. Davidson, *The Marketing Sourcebook for Small Business* (New York: John Wiley & Sons, Inc., 1989), 101.

3. L. Sachs, *Do-It-Yourself Marketing for the Professional Practice* (Englewood Cliffs, N.J.: Prentice-Hall, Inc., 1986), 78.

4. MacStravic, "Professional and Personal Quality of Care in Health Care Delivery," 64.

chapter 5

Selling

Although the concepts of marketing, public relations, and even advertising are gaining acceptance as necessary ways to inform the health care consumer of the advantages of one organization over another, selling remains an anathema to many health care professionals. *Webster's Dictionary* lists eight definitions of the word sell. Five of these definitions hold negative connotations, such as "betray," "cheat," "to give up in return for something else especially foolishly or dishonorably," "to deliver into slavery for money," and "to dispose of or manage for profit instead of in accordance with conscience, justice, or duty."[1] The other three definitions are simply neutral, such as "to influence to a course of action" and "to cause or promote sale of." It is no wonder that health care professionals, who are trained to promote the higher good of humanity, often have trouble recognizing and admitting that selling may be a positive and beneficial activity for themselves, their organizations, and consumers. When performed honestly and ethically, however, selling is an honorable activity that informs, supports, and provides service benefits to the consumer while directly increasing an organization's market share, improving the organization's bottom line, and helping to deal effectively with the competition. Selling is an appropriate part of the marketing mix that can establish and maintain customer satisfaction, positive word-of-mouth promotions, and repeat business.

Kotler and Clarke describe three types of salespersons: the order taker, the order getter, and the customer need satisfier.[2] The order taker is too passive; this salesperson believes that customers already know what they need, that they would resent any attempt to influence them, and that they prefer self-effacing salespersons. The order getter, on the other hand, is too aggressive. The order getter believes that customers will not buy without a hard sell and slick presentations; moreover, the order getter does not care if customers are displeased with the sale. The third type of salesperson, the customer need satisfier, believes that customers may need assistance in defining their needs in relation to the organization's benefits. The customer need satisfier believes that customers "appreciate good suggestions and . . . they will be responsive to representatives who have their interests at heart."[3]

PERSONAL SELLING

In personal selling, there is a one-on-one interaction between a representative of an organization with a product or service to sell and a prospective customer with a need that may be met by the product or service offered. The critical feature of this type of selling is its personal nature, which provides an opportunity for the salesperson to build a relationship with a prospect prior to obtaining a commitment to purchase. The prospect, that is, the potential consumer, can obtain tangible evidence of the organization's service qualities through the demeanor, presentation, and attitude of the salesperson.

As global politics are being transformed and previous military enemies are learning to live side by side to their mutual benefit, so it is in selling on a personal level. The adversarial, warlike approach in which someone wins and someone loses no longer works in selling. The military concept in marketing is being replaced by relationship-building customer satisfaction and value provision. Even in commercial and service sales, such as retail and hotels, a transition is occurring in which the customer-driven, cooperative salesperson who believes in win-win resolutions to mutual problems is replacing the dominant, aggressive salesperson who functions and thinks in militaristic terms. The concepts of beating down objections and closing the sale are transformed in this newer approach into concepts of "educating and informing the buyer" and "bringing the buyer to yes." Rather than creating an adversarial sales climate, the modern salesperson forms an alliance with the buyer to provide information that facilitates decision making, trust, and a partnership that develops over time.

The focus of relationship building in personal selling is on long-term commitment and repeat sales. This approach takes into account the fact that the buying decision is based on more than logic and perceived need. Emotions play a role for the buyer in determining the value of the purchase. The salesperson who is positioned as a "consultant" to the buyer recognizes the need to be trustworthy and representative of a product that is service- and customer-driven and that the product must live up to the quality described by the salesperson to ensure repeat purchases.

Benefits of Personal Selling

Three unique benefits are added to the marketing mix through personal selling.

1. face-to-face interaction
2. relationship-building opportunity
3. prospect response

A face-to-face interaction is a powerful way to personalize an organization's message. The personal interview or sales call gives tangibility and credibility to the organization's message and attributes. Sales calls also provide the salesperson with an opportunity to build a personal/professional relationship with the potential consumer. Once the consumer realizes that the salesperson's promises are backed up by the organization's service record, credibility, and trust, a long-term relationship has begun.

The third benefit of personal selling is that the prospect must respond in some way to the personal interaction. Even if the response is negative, the salesperson may obtain information that can benefit the organization's future marketing efforts. Other, less personal forms of marketing allow for a nonresponse, which can mean many things from ''no, not ever,'' to ''not just now, thank you.'' The immediate verbal and nonverbal feedback inherent in personal selling provides richer, more valuable information to the organization.

Similarity of Personal Selling to Physical Therapy

Physical therapists use sales skills from the beginning of their first job. From interviewing for the job to persuading a supervisor or administrator to approve a budget increase, a staffing increase, the purchase of new equipment, or space allocation, the therapist engages in personal sales activities. Persuading a physician to change a treatment protocol on a patient care plan requires successful selling of the treatment plan to the physician. Discussing the services and benefits offered by the clinic with a potential referral source, such as a business, a physician, or a managed care group, is a selling activity. Persuading patients of the importance of participating in a home exercise program often requires great sales skills. All of these scenarios demonstrate how physical therapists successfully perform one-on-one personal selling every single day.

Because simply being a competent physical therapist often takes great sales ability, physical therapists have developed many of the selling skills that are necessary for success. Six traits separate great salespersons from mediocre ones, and physical therapists exhibit all six of these skills.

1. care about service
2. care about the customer
3. empathy with the customer
4. image

5. active listening
6. awareness of the importance of repetition and persistence

Perhaps the similarities between great salespersons and physical therapists come from the fact that they both are in the communication business; these traits are evidenced by those who have learned to be good communicators.

It is important for physical therapists to remember that they already possess the six traits that make great salespersons when performing a one-on-one sales call. They should tell the prospect that service is their business and let their enthusiasm show. They should make it obvious that they care about the patients and clients that come to them; they should tell several stories about patients' satisfaction with their services in the past. During the sales call, it is always essential to listen actively to the prospect in order to find out what is important to him or her about physical therapy services. Finally, it will probably be necessary to repeat the message five or six times before the prospect will feel comfortable enough to refer patients to the clinic.

Sales Calls

The traditional sales call occurs in the office of a prospect after an appointment has been made. The prospect may be any target market, including the potential or current referring physician, a business or industry executive who wants to buy a physical therapy program or service, a hospital administrator who wants to contract for physical therapy services, or an insurance company representative who makes decisions regarding insurance reimbursement policies. Sales calls need not be limited to appointed, prearranged meetings, however. A brief sales call format used during a chance encounter with a physician in a hospital hallway or during a social occasion can be effective as well. The process of probing to determine the wants and needs of target markets, listing the clinic's benefits as they pertain to the prospect's perceptions, and keeping the needs and goals of the clinic in mind is an effective way to build long-term relationships with a target market.

Purpose of a Sales Call

Sales calls have five purposes.

1. selling
2. informing
3. obtaining new customers
4. following up service
5. researching the market

Although the primary purpose is to make a sale, the four other objectives may also be met. In fact, most sales calls are made with a mix of these objectives in mind.

A therapist should rank the importance of each specific objective of a sales call in order to maintain the focus of the call. The appropriate priority depends to a great extent on where the prospect is in the hierarchy of effects. For example, the objectives of informing, researching the market, and obtaining new customers would rank high in a sales call to a prospect who has only just learned of the availability of the clinic's service, while the objectives of selling and following up service would have a lower priority in such a call. On the other hand, the reverse would be the case in a sales call on a customer who has used the service previously. Each of these sales objectives should be recognized, given a priority, and rewarded by the organization.

Making an Appointment

Many people have difficulty setting up a sales call by telephone. They should begin by stating their name and the reason that they would like to meet. For example, "Hello, I am Kay Schaefer from Physical Therapy Health Center. We have several unique features that we think can benefit you and your patients. I need about twenty minutes of your time." This statement should be followed by a double positive in order to elicit the desired response, such as "Is Tuesday morning or Thursday morning okay? Would 10 or 10:30 be better?" This gives the prospect a choice of two answers, either of which is acceptable to the clinic representative and neither of which is "no."

It is important to be persistent, but always to be polite, positive, and friendly. Furthermore, it is always helpful to get the name of the secretary or receptionist and use it on the next call.

Preparation for a Sales Call

Effective sales calls begin with significant preparation. The first step is image preparation. The therapist lists the adjectives that describe the image that honestly and professionally represents the clinic's service and its benefits (see Chapter 3). Then the therapist should review what is known about the prospect and the prospect's company in order to match his or her personal professional image to the prospect's expectations. Then the therapist matches his or her appearance and presentation style as a clinic representative with the prospect's expectations (Exhibit 5-1).

It is also important to determine where the prospect is in the hierarchy of effects in order to establish sales potential (Exhibit 5-2). When the prospect has never been exposed to the clinic previously, the first sales call is the first impression. As mentioned earlier, the purpose of the sales call in this case is simply to obtain name recognition for future marketing interactions. If the prospect has worked with the

Exhibit 5-1 Image Preparation for a Sales Call

Image Adjectives That Describe Service Benefits and Physical Therapy	Prospect's Expectations	Therapist's Appearance and Presentation Style
_____	_____	_____
_____	_____	_____
_____	_____	_____
_____	_____	_____
_____	_____	_____
_____	_____	_____
_____	_____	_____
_____	_____	_____
_____	_____	_____
_____	_____	_____
_____	_____	_____

clinic previously, the message will need to be different. Follow-up sales calls to regular customers are essential to monitor satisfaction and to encourage repeat use.

The therapist on a sales call must know the needs of the prospect, must always keep them in mind, and must be constantly ready to revise those needs as is appropriate during the sales call. Because a successful salesperson is a consultant to the prospect, most of the effort should be spent on determining the prospects' needs and tailoring the presentation to those needs. The focus must be kept on the customer and the customer's business, particularly as it relates to the clinic. Although a prepared presentation is essential, the therapist must be equally prepared to change that presentation as the conversation requires.

If possible, the therapist should determine the prospect's needs before the sales call in order to start out with a competitive edge (Exhibit 5-3). For example, in preparing for a sales call to a referring internist, the therapist may call the secretary to ask where the internist sends patients for physical therapy now and if he or she is satisfied. The secretary may say, "As a matter of fact, sending our patients to an orthopedic surgeon causes my boss to lose contact with patients." Given this

Exhibit 5-2 Hierarchy of Effects: Prospect Position

☐ 1. Unawareness	☐ 6. Decision
☐ 2. Awareness	☐ 7. Satisfaction
☐ 3. Understanding	☐ 8. Repeat use
☐ 4. Familiarity	☐ 9. Recommendation
☐ 5. Interest	

information, the therapist now knows how best to target the comments to the internist. The clinic can meet at least one of the internist's needs by guaranteeing patients' return for follow-up, which puts the clinic at an advantage. Once the sales call begins, the therapist can ask enough questions to determine additional needs, such as what type of patients the internist sees primarily and how the internist perceives the benefits of physical therapy. The answers to open-ended questions like these (i.e., questions that require more than a ''yes'' or ''no'' response) will indicate whether the internist has established referral practices or may be willing to refer patients to a new clinic.

In preparing for the sales call, the therapist must learn the benefits of the clinic's product (service) backward and forward by outcome. The new Cybex unit is *not* a benefit of the clinic's product. This expensive piece of technology must be translated into an outcome benefit for the prospect. For example, if the prospect is an orthopedic surgeon, the therapist may discuss how rehabilitation time has decreased and patient satisfaction has increased since the clinic purchased a Cybex unit. A prospect will not necessarily make the link between those things that are of

Exhibit 5-3 Target Market Needs Research

Before the Sales Call	*Response*
1. Ask the secretary.	_____
2. Ask the prospect.	_____
3. Ask colleagues, physicians and physical therapists.	_____
During the Sales Call	
1. Note verbal feedback to open-ended questions.	_____
2. Note nonverbal feedback.	_____

significance to the clinic and a patient's needs. The clinic's benefits must be described in terms of a solution to the prospect's problems.

The therapist should prepare a notebook with support materials to take along during the sales call. Such a notebook indicates preparedness and is a tangible reflection of the clinic or service. It should contain items such as the clinic's brochure, news articles, proposals, referral pad, giveaways, sample forms/letters, and newsletters.

Once the therapist is fully prepared for the sales call, it is time to practice. Many people who are new to selling need at least three practice sessions at first. Some therapists like to practice in front of a mirror so that they can determine their facial expressions and recognize their nonverbal communications.

On the way to the sales call, it may be helpful to repeat positive thoughts, such as ''This presentation will go well,'' ''My objectives will be reached,'' and ''I am enthusiastic about my clinic.'' Simple positive sayings such as this truly affect a therapist's mood and ability to make a relaxed, successful presentation. Exhibit 5-4 is a summary of sales call preparation.

Exhibit 5-4 Sales Calls: Preparation

1. Describe the image you wish to project.
   _____   _____

2. Where is the prospect in the hierarchy of effects?
   ☐ Unawareness   ☐ Decision
   ☐ Awareness   ☐ Satisfaction
   ☐ Familiarity   ☐ Repeat use
   ☐ Understanding

3. List the prospect's wants and needs as they relate to your service.
   _____
   _____

4. List potential open-ended questions based on the purpose of the sales call as previously determined.
   _____
   _____

5. List your product's benefits in terms that address the prospect's wants and needs.
   _____
   _____

6. Bring support materials.
   ☐ Brochure   ☐ Referral pad
   ☐ Sample forms   ☐ Giveaways
   ☐ Sample letters   ☐ Newsletter

7. Practice.
   _____ To self
   _____ To friend or colleague
   _____ To mirror

The Sales Call Itself

Just as a good book has an opening, a body, and a closing, so does a successful sales call (Exhibit 5-5). The optimal amount of time for a sales call is generally in the range of twenty minutes. It is important to be flexible, however, in order to take advantage of whatever amount of personal interaction time is available.

Opening. The sales call opening is the initial greeting between the therapist and the prospect. During this greeting, the therapist should keep enthusiastic, keep relaxed, and keep a positive attitude to make a good first impression. Rapport can be established quickly in no more than one or two sentences. During the opening, the therapist may present one to three major product benefits. If the prospect is a physician, for example, the therapist may highlight the fact that (1) the clinic sends an initial evaluation to the physician within twenty-four hours of seeing the patient for the first time, (2) the patient returns to the physician at the time of discharge, and (3) the clinic has a no waiting policy. The therapist should observe the prospect's reactions, both verbal and nonverbal, for areas to probe later during the body of the sales call. Also during the opening, the therapist should be sure to state the meeting goals, such as to "explain our service so that you feel confident sending patients to us." Finally, the therapist should get feedback during the opening concerning the prospect's reaction to the three benefits and the meeting goals. It is important to ask questions and confirm nonverbal body language and facial expressions. The opening should be brief, lasting only two to five minutes.

Exhibit 5-5 The Sales Call

Opening	*Closing*
• Be enthusiastic	• Summarize benefits
• Establish rapport	• Get a commitment
• Present 1 to 3 product benefits	• If refused: Stay enthusiastic
• State your meeting goals	Don't take it personally
• Be aware of feedback	• If accepted: Reinforce prospect's decision
	Let prospect end meeting
Body	
• Use support materials	
• Base presentation on feedback	
• Ask open-ended questions	
• Discuss benefits from prospect's point of view	

Body. During the body of the sales call, which takes the most amount of time, the therapist uses the support materials to follow up on the product benefits in which the prospect showed an interest during the opening. Although it is important during this stage to ask questions, it is also important to stay in control and not let the discussion stray from the purpose. This can be difficult without interrupting or appearing rude, but practice will bring finesse in this skill. It may be helpful to watch how reporters keep interviews on track. A prospect should never be cut off in mid-sentence, but it may be possible to find a thread in the current topic to bring the conversation back on target.

The body of the sales call is the time for greater in-depth discussion of the benefits of the clinic's services and further efforts to probe the prospect's reaction to the benefits. Open-ended questions can be used to elicit additional feedback. For example, the therapist may ask the internist, "What are the three most important considerations for you when you select a physical therapy clinic to send your patients?" This open-ended question is designed to elicit opinions, attitudes, and beliefs that not only may direct the rest of the sales call, but also may provide valuable information about the marketplace. If one of the internist's considerations matches a benefit that the therapist stated in the opening, the therapist should offer more information about this benefit.

Open-ended questions such as "What would you like to see changed about the way that most clinics provide physical therapy?" are designed to reveal objections or obstacles that may be preventing the prospect from sending patients to the clinic. Knowing the objections provides the therapist with an opportunity to clarify and overcome them or to admit that the objection may be a true barrier to usage and a change in the clinic's organizational structure may be necessary. Either way, an honest response that accepts the possibility of shortcomings in the clinic's service or explains alternatives within the existing system will lay the groundwork for a potential long-term relationship by demonstrating flexibility and adaptability to outside conditions.

During the body of the sales call, the therapist must remember to discuss the product's benefits in terms related to the prospect's wants and needs. Instead of emphasizing the advanced training of the staff in terms of the number of seminars that they have attended and the instructors with whom they have studied, the therapist should emphasize the qualitative difference in patient outcome associated with a staff that have advanced training and skills. The story or case study approach can drive the point home. For example, "Before obtaining advanced training, our average number of patient visits for the diagnosis was twelve. Now, after the training, we are averaging seven patient visits for the same diagnosis. Patients are back to work much sooner."

Closing. When the therapist has made the three major points and has answered the prospect's questions, it is time for the closing. Once again, the therapist should summarize the three major product benefits, as the closing is the opportunity to get a commitment. The meeting goal can be rephrased as a question; for example, "Have I explained our services so that you feel confident in sending patients to us?" If the prospect refuses, the therapist should stay enthusiastic and should not take the refusal personally. The real reason for the refusal may have nothing to do with the therapist or the clinic. If the therapist remains enthusiastic while being refused, however, opportunities remain open for the future. If during the closing the prospect accepts the proposal and agrees to send patients to the clinic, the therapist should reinforce the prospect's decision by expressing appreciation and let the prospect end the meeting.

Follow-Up and Evaluation

The sales call must be followed up by sending a letter that restates comments made during the meeting. Pertinent information, such as a recent clinic newsletter or article reprint that pertains to the conversation, should be included. If it is appropriate, a follow-up telephone call may be made to answer a question or clarify a point discussed during the meeting.

As with all marketing efforts, the effectiveness of sales calls must be evaluated. If the primary purpose of the call was to increase referrals, the referral patterns of the prospects before and after the sales call should be tracked. If the purpose was to change an insurance company's reimbursement policy, it is necessary to check periodically to determine if the change has been made. If part of the purpose was to research the market, a file of market information gathered through sales calls should be maintained. A lead sheet or a sales call report should be used to list all the calls that have been made and what happened during each call (Exhibit 5-6). The objective of the call, the results, the follow-up action, and the results of the follow-up should be documented. Regular evaluation is as important to sales call outcome as it is to patient care outcome in physical therapy.

Costs

Sales calls are a relatively expensive form of marketing because they are labor-intensive. In 1982, a physician sales call by a pharmaceutical representative cost $75.[4] The cost of the sales calls made for a physical therapy clinic includes preparation time, time to arrange the meeting, travel time, actual sales time, and follow-up time. Materials must also be taken into consideration, as well as the salary and benefits of the person who made the sales call. If that person is a physical therapist, the revenue lost because the therapist was not treating patients during that time must also be included.

In spite of the expense, the benefits of performing targeted sales calls often outweigh the costs. Physical therapy is a personalized service that can be effectively promoted and made tangible through a personal sales call.

Exhibit 5-6 Sales Call Report

Prospect Name	Date	Objectives	Results	Follow-Up	Results

Cold Call Selling

An unannounced visit to a prospect's office is an approach referred to as cold call selling. Few professionals have unfilled moments and a cold call may be considered an intrusion. Few professionals object, however, if the salesperson is stopping by to drop off a business card and make an appointment. The impression under those circumstances is slightly stronger than that made by a telephone call, but it is an expensive way to make an appointment. For the time that cold call selling requires, the return in terms of actual selling time is relatively small. Nevertheless, in many physicians' offices, the nurse or receptionist makes the referral decision, and a cold call may be worthwhile in these offices. Using the skills of a sales call with all decision makers in an office, including the receptionist, enhances the return on investment.

Cold calls may be strategically advantageous in the market plan of a new clinic. Because the clinic is not well-known in the community, its representatives may find it more difficult to make appointments, and a series of cold calls will help increase the clinic's visibility. Cold calls may also be appropriate if a therapist wants to enter new markets, expand the business, or periodically visit a large number of referral sources to get a feel for market changes. As with all marketing efforts, it is essential to determine the organizational goal to be accomplished, the image to be projected, and the point of view of the prospect before initiating a cold call selling campaign. It is also critical to evaluate the effectiveness of such a campaign.

TELECOMMUNICATIONS: SELLING BY TELEPHONE

The telephone is a powerful marketing tool. It is cost-effective because it is a personal one-on-one interaction with the target market without the time or expense of a personal sales call. Any telephone call is an opportunity to communicate a message verbally.

Strategies for Telecommunications

There are two strategies for telecommunications: (1) turning every telephone call into a marketing effort and (2) performing prepared sales communications by telephone. The first approach requires very little additional expenditure of time and provides excellent results. For example, if the clinic has just purchased a new piece of equipment, such as an iontophoresis unit, for the next week or two staff members can tag a little informational sales pitch onto the end of all their conversations with referring physicians when they discuss patient care. After discussing the evaluation of Mrs. Smith's condition with Dr. Jones, the therapist can state, "By the way, we just purchased a new iontophoresis unit. Tendonitis and bursitis generally respond well to treatment with this unit. The three major benefits of iontophoresis are that it is (1) noninvasive, (2) locally administered, and (3) virtually pain-free." These statements can be followed with a brief description of the unit and its use: "Iontophoresis uses electrical current to push hydrocortisone molecules through the skin and into the inflamed area, covering an area that is about an inch in diameter. Since we have been using this unit, we have had excellent results in the reduction of pain, as well as in early mobilization and strengthening of the tissue involved, without any need for an injection or oral medication." It takes about a minute to make that explanation and determine where in the hierarchy of effects this physician is positioned concerning iontophoresis and the possibility of his sending patients to the clinic.

If the physician is interested, the therapist can send a previously prepared follow-up letter that restates the description of iontophoresis, its major benefits, and the type of injuries for which it works best, as well as a successful case study.

In addition, the therapist may send one or two reprints of an article on the use of iontophoresis. The clinic's secretary can fill in the physician's name and send the prepared package.

A major benefit of this approach is that it is a tremendous time-saver. It takes approximately twenty minutes to prepare the basic telephone communication for the physician and thirty to forty-five minutes to prepare the standard follow-up letter and packet. This preparation time is spread over all the physicians actually contacted. It takes approximately five minutes to make the sales pitch on the telephone and mail the packet. For this effort, the clinic's sales message has two exposures to the target market—one by telephone and the second by letter.

Physical therapists can also use telecommunications to market their services through prepared telephone selling messages to a specified list of potential consumers. They can use this approach to set a date for a personal sales call, to familiarize the target market with their product, to establish satisfaction levels, to determine new needs, or to encourage repeat use. The first thing that they must do in using this technique, however, is to overcome any fear that they have in performing the telephone sales call. Many people fear that they will say the wrong thing, communicate the message poorly, make a bad impression, or end with a negative rather than a positive outcome from the telephone call. The best way to overcome these fears is through practice, both alone and with a friend. Second, they must prepare not only the content of the telephone call, but also the image that they wish to promote with their tone of voice, their persuasiveness, their choice of words, and their overall professionalism.

Three Steps in Successful Telecommunications

The three steps in a successful telecommunications effort are (1) preparation, (2) performance, and (3) follow-up (Exhibit 5-7).

Exhibit 5-7 Three Steps in Successful Telecommunications

1. *Preparation*	• Listen for response
• Determine target market	• Modify contents
• List purpose	• Summarize
• Prepare support documents	
	3. *Follow-Up*
2. *Performance*	• Do what you promise
• Make beginning statement	
• Be concise	

Preparation

Preparing the telecommunications effort in advance allows therapists to use their contact time most effectively. Preparation includes determining who the target market will be and what motivates the target market to want, need, and use physical therapy. The purpose of the call and the expected outcome in relation to the clinic's strategic plan and marketing goals should be listed. Support documents, including a copy of the opening statement, an outline of the conversation, a list of the three benefits to communicate, and a benefits statement that may be used to attain the objective of the communication, should be readily available during the call. The call should be made in a quiet place where there will be no interruptions.

Performance

The beginning statement creates a lasting impression. The therapist should speak clearly and precisely in a friendly tone of voice. Literally smiling while speaking helps project a warm sincere attitude, which the other party can detect. The therapist should get the message across in the first twenty seconds and then listen for the prospect's response in order to tailor additional comments and benefit statements to that response. At the end of the call, the therapist not only should summarize the contents and mutually expected outcome, but also should state the time and method of the follow-up contact. This may be a personal visit or the mailing of information and support materials.

Follow-Up

Once the telecommunications effort has been completed, follow-up is extremely important. It is essential to follow through with anything that was promised during the telephone call, including a follow-up letter, literature, a subsequent telephone call, or a meeting that may have been planned.

DIRECT MAIL MARKETING

Many organizations undertake a direct mail marketing campaign in which they mail promotional pieces to a specifically targeted population for the purpose of obtaining a response. Common forms of direct mail in physical therapy include newsletters, brochures, and promotional letters designed to catch the attention of the reader and create a desire to take some action. In order to trigger the action, the direct mail piece must clearly address a need of the recipient. The targeted consumer benefits should be placed at the beginning of the direct mail piece so that the reader can readily understand the reason to take action. The action statement, which requests the reader to obtain information or a benefit by making a call, sending in a reply, redeeming a coupon, or attending a function (e.g., an open house), is placed near the end of the piece. The response rate indicates the success of the direct mail piece; a 3 percent to 5 percent response rate for a direct mail marketing campaign is considered good.[5]

Benefits of Direct Mail Marketing

A recent U.S. Postal Service survey found that people open and read 78 percent of the promotional material that they receive in the mail.[6] People read mail in their homes at a time of their own choosing, thus making direct mail personal and convenient. Although it must be considered when marketing with direct mail, the negative image of "junk mail" can be overcome through the design and copy aspects of the piece. Direct mail looks less like junk mail when the address is typed directly on the envelope rather than appearing through a cellophane window or even on a mailing label. Colored paper may catch the reader's attention, but yellows and pinks on thin weight paper suggest the more commercial and cheaper junk mail. Grey, eggshell, and dusty blue present a more formal, professional, and less commercial image.

Direct mail may be the marketing tool of choice for targeting a specific market segment demographically or geographically. For example, as demographic mailing lists can be age-specific, a functional independence program designed for the elderly may be marketed directly to potential users of the service, as well as to their adult children. A direct mail piece emphasizing continued self-reliance and independence can be sent to people aged seventy to ninety years; a piece emphasizing the peace of mind that an adult child wants in the safety of a parent living alone can be sent to people aged forty to fifty years. This specificity of target audience is a very important advantage of direct mail advertising.

Geographic mailing can also differentiate between ZIP codes that are primarily industrial and those that are primarily residential. It can even indicate average household income. In the example mentioned, mailings would not be sent to business ZIP codes, but rather to residential areas in order to target individuals more likely to use the service. The residential areas can be broken down even further to target the higher income families that are more likely to have discretionary income for an elderly day care service.

Mailing List

The key to successful direct mail marketing is a clean mailing list. Such a list has no incorrect addresses, is culled of people who have moved, and is made up almost exclusively of individuals who are likely to purchase the product or service. It has been said that "you can send a mediocre package to a good mailing list and achieve better results than by sending a great package to a poor mailing list."[7] This remark emphasizes the strategic significance of a clean mailing list. Obtaining a clean mailing list is one of the most difficult aspects of direct mail marketing, however. Mailing lists must be updated frequently to be clean and targeted for marketing efforts geared toward the repeat user and satisfied customer.

There are two primary ways to obtain a mailing list: (1) by developing it in-house from past, current, and potential customers and (2) by purchasing it from a list broker. Physical therapy clinics have information bases that make it possible to develop lists of physicians, patients, and insurance carriers. A physician list can specify for each referring physician the specialty, address, telephone number, dominant insurance type, number of patients referred per month, and average number of visits per referred patient (Exhibit 5-8). This mailing list can be updated

---

Exhibit 5-8 Physician Mailing List

Physician Name and Specialty	Address	Telephone Number	Dominant Insurance Type	Number Patients Referred	Visits per Referred Patient

monthly with new referral sources, address corrections, and deletions of obsolete names. Mailing lists can also be compiled of physicians who are potential referral sources from the local American Medical Association's *Physician Directory*, the Yellow Pages, or the lists of physicians on staff at local hospitals. It is also a good idea to keep a list of the names, addresses, and payment methods of satisfied patients. Returned patient satisfaction surveys and the opinions of the physical therapists on staff may be used to compile this list (Exhibit 5-9).

In addition to physicians and patients, insurance carriers may be a target market worth direct mail marketing (Exhibit 5-10). With changing reimbursement methods, it may be an advantageous marketing strategy for a physical therapy clinic to stay visible to the policy makers and claims adjusters at private insurance companies, as well as health maintenance organizations, preferred provider organizations, and independent provider organizations. This mailing list may include the

---

Exhibit 5-9 Patient Mailing List

Patient Name	Address	Telephone Number	Payment Method	Year Treated

Exhibit 5-10 Insurance Company Mailing List

Insurance Carrier Name	*Key Contact People*	*Job Title*	*Physical Therapy Payment Policies*	*Attitudinal Trends*

name and position of key contacts at the insurance company and their payment policies regarding in-house physical therapy.

List brokers can be found in the Yellow Pages or through local professional public relations firms, advertising agencies, and firms that specialize in direct mail marketing. List brokers function through computers that hook up to mailing lists from across the United States. Some list brokers specialize in consumer lists; some, in business and industry lists. Although the fees of list brokers are essentially similar, the quality of their lists varies according to their in-house methods of address verification, list merging, and list purging. If possible, it may be wise to ask for recommendations concerning any list broker considered. Large lists usually cost between $15 to $100 per thousand names.[8] In general, the smaller, more specific, and cleaner lists are more costly per name than are larger lists. Benefits and disadvantages of direct mail advertising are listed in Exhibit 5-11.

Exhibit 5-11 Advantages and Disadvantages of Direct Mail Advertising

Advantages	Disadvantages
• Personalized to the target audience	• Possible association with junk mail
• Convenience for the reader	• Clean mailing list sometimes difficult to obtain
• Specific demographic and geographic targeting	
• Control over mailing list	

Development of a Direct Mail Marketing Campaign

Although a sophisticated direct mail campaign is best performed by a firm that specializes in such campaigns, there are many direct mail marketing activities that can be performed in-house successfully. These include regular newsletter mailings, open house or event mailings, and standard letters to potential or new referral sources. Large groups of potential consumers or physicians may best be targeted through a direct mail firm.

The first step in developing a direct mail campaign is to determine its objective and the way in which it fits into the organization's strategic plan. Knowing the desired outcome of this marketing activity makes its effectiveness measurable. Before developing the promotional piece, it is necessary to review the physical therapy clinic's position in the marketplace, its differential advantage, and the perceived place of the target market in the hierarchy of effects. This review ensures that the direct mail piece will be consistent with other organizational marketing efforts. The design of the marketing piece should be coordinated with related messages in terms of logo, color, and overall appearance.

A primary concern is that the piece should address the business or personal needs of the prospect rather than those of the clinic. In reading the literature, the prospect will be asking, "What's in it for me?" That question should be answered in the first sentence or paragraph. Highlighting the benefits to the prospect in the beginning of the piece encourages the prospect to read further, to use the service, or to respond to the direct mail piece.

A direct mail piece should also include an incentive for the prospect to take responsive action. In physical therapy, as in most types of health care, giving away free information is a good incentive. A toll-free 800 number, a response card, or both may be used to stimulate action. The information given away may be in the form of a brochure, a letter, or a newsletter. Providing free information establishes the clinic's staff as experts in the field and enhances their credibility. The response rate must be measured to establish the effectiveness of the direct mail piece.

Respondents also can be added to mailing lists as quality prospects. The ten steps in developing a direct mail campaign are listed in Exhibit 5-12.

Direct mail marketing must be part of an overall marketing strategy. One mailing of one piece to a target audience cannot achieve a marketing objective. This marketing tool is very versatile, however, and may be used with a target market at any stage of the hierarchy of effects.

Other marketing strategies coordinate well with direct mailings. The best strategies involve several mailings, at least four to six weeks apart, with telecommunications marketing as a follow-up with the prospects. When appropriate, sales calls may be made to follow up the most promising leads. As in all marketing efforts, it is essential to offer only that which can be delivered and to deliver more than is promised in order to ensure satisfaction and success in direct mail advertising.

Exhibit 5-12 Steps in Developing a Direct Mail Campaign

1. Determine the objective of this direct mail campaign.

2. State the organization's strategic goal for this campaign.

3. How will the effectiveness of this campaign be measured?

4. Review the organization's position in the marketplace.

5. Review the clinic's differential advantage.

6. Identify the target market and its position in the hierarchy of effects.

7. Review logo, color, overall message, and look with other marketing pieces and the organization's image to achieve a coordinated effort.

8. Does the direct mail piece answer the prospect's question ''What's in it for me?'' in the first sentence or paragraph?

9. State the incentive for the prospect to take further action.

10. Measure effectiveness through response rate.

NOTES

1. *Webster's Ninth New Collegiate Dictionary* (Springfield, Mass.: Merriam-Webster, Inc., 1984).

2. P. Kotler and R.N. Clarke, *Marketing for Health Care Organizations* (Englewood Cliffs, N.J.: Prentice-Hall, Inc., 1987), 416–417.

3. Ibid., 417.

4. Ibid., 405.

5. W.J. Winston, ed., *Advertising Handbook for Health Care Services* (New York: The Haworth Press, Inc., 1986), 21.

6. Physician's Marketing Kit, Physician's Marketing.

7. C. Ryan, *Strategies To Market Smarter in the 90's*. Remarks to the Direct Marketing Association of Washington, March 1990.

8. R.S. MacStravic, "Professional and Personal Quality of Care in Health Care Delivery," *Health Marketing Quarterly* 5 (1987/88): 290–309.

chapter *6*

Advertising

One of the marketing tools used to implement a marketing strategy is advertising. It differs from other tools as a promotional activity in that an organization pays for it directly. Strategically combined in the marketing mix with internal marketing, public relations, and selling, advertising completes a promotional package for a marketing objective.

GROWTH OF HEALTH CARE ADVERTISING

The acceptance of health care advertising, initiated after the elimination of legal restraints by a U.S. Supreme Court ruling in 1977,[1] has been slow. Health care professionals, facilities, and professional associations have voiced concern that advertising may lead consumers into purchasing costly health care that they may not want or need. Nevertheless, health care advertising is becoming more common—not only because of increasing competition in the health care field for the consumer's dollar, but also because of a sincere desire to inform the public about the availability and benefits of services.

As health care advertising comes out of its infancy and moves into adolescence, it is experiencing many growing pains. These growing pains have taught an expensive lesson to many health care institutions. Some institutions have advertised for a while, then stopped advertising, and then sometimes advertised in a haphazard or spotty fashion without any apparent plan. This has occurred primarily because of top executives' failure to understand the advertising function and the large expense incurred by advertising. Many administrators had unrealistic expectations of an advertising campaign and often decided to advertise based solely on the observation that the competition was advertising. When, after a year or so of advertising, the health care advertiser was not able to identify a direct return on investment for advertising dollars spent, advertising campaigns often were withdrawn. These health care executives were slow to realize that advertising is a long-term commitment and that advertising outcome can rarely be measured in revenue during the short term.

Advertising campaigns are staged to bring the target market through the hierarchy of effects. Therefore, the goal of introductory advertising is often simply name recognition. Outcome is measured by population surveys before and after the campaign. The next advertising strategy is often an image campaign, designed simply to familiarize the market with an organization's service benefits. The third campaign in this ongoing series may be designed to foster a decision to use the service. The market may be encouraged to respond to this campaign by calling a toll-free 800 number or stopping by the facility to pick up free information or a free screening service; the response rate measures the effectiveness of this campaign. The next advertising strategy may focus on various product lines offered by the organization in order to generate increased volume sales. Depending on the community, the competition, the marketing strategy, and the budget, this process may take six months to several years to complete.

Because physical therapists as a group and as individuals have not yet done much advertising, they can learn valuable lessons from the experience of other health care organizations. The use of advertising in the marketing mix must be well thought out and must fit into the organization's strategic plan, as well as into the coordinated marketing plan. Product marketers recognize that television or radio advertising, particularly of a new product or a product that is not understood or well-known by the general public, requires significant exposure and repetition to be successful. A consumer must be exposed to an advertisement message "three to six times before any significant positioning occurs in the minds of the target groups."[2] The average consumer is exposed to more than 1,200 advertisements per day and, therefore, unconsciously picks and chooses those worthy of remembering.[3] It has also been found that the average consumer forgets more than half of these messages within an hour.[4] In advertising, an organization must break through this information clutter; its advertising must be unique, creative, and related to the needs of the advertising audience.

In addition, advertising must take into account the position of the target audience in the hierarchy of effects. For example, McDonald's recognizes that most people are familiar with their product and immediately envision a hamburger when they see the name McDonald's or the golden arches. Therefore, their advertising is aimed at satisfaction, repeat use, and recommendation of their product. McDonald's commercials now feature humorous or touching human interest stories that reach the emotion of the potential repeat user. McDonald's understood its target market's position in the hierarchy of effects. Physical therapists must also recognize at the planning stages where consumers are in the hierarchy of effects in order to target advertising specifically to their interest level and informational needs.

BENEFITS OF ADVERTISING

As mentioned earlier, many health care professionals have false expectations about advertising; they believe that, because the cost is so high, it should immediately translate into increased profits. Advertising is a long-term commitment that positions the product or service over years of repeated exposure, however; it does not produce instant results, and it requires money.

Although it is essential to plan carefully prior to embarking on an advertising campaign, advertising does offer unique promotional advantages (Exhibit 6-1). It exposes a program to major segments of the population. The media, including television, radio, newspaper, and magazines, all offer tremendous exposure to a large portion of the general population. This widespread exposure is almost impossible to obtain except through advertising.

Advertising also allows an organization to control the message, timing, content, and dimensions of the exposure to the general public. Because the clinic is paying for the message, the staff can choose the exact content of the message and the benefits of the clinic to be highlighted. Additionally, because the staff controls the time of the year and the time of the day that the advertisement will run, they can target the small segment of the population that is likely to respond to the advertising.

The advertising director of any medium in which an advertisement is to run can recommend a time and placement for the advertisement that will give the desired subsegment of the target population maximum exposure to the message. For example, if the advertisement is designed to appeal to the elderly, it is well-known that the elderly watch television primarily during the early evening hours; some segments of the elderly market also listen to radio programs in the middle of the night because they have difficulty sleeping. Newspaper advertising directors know which segments of the paper are best for particular advertisements. For example, an advertisement for a sports medicine clinic obviously belongs on the sports page. On the other hand, the newspaper advertising director may share the information that people who are interested in recreational sports also read the financial section of the newspaper and that advertising space in the financial section is less expensive than is advertising space in the sports section.

Exhibit 6-1 Advantages and Disadvantages of Advertising

Advantages	*Disadvantages*
• Exposure to large and specifically targeted segments of the population • Control over message, timing, and content	• Cost • Long-term commitment

Adults between the ages of thirty-five and forty-nine pay attention to advertisements that are fun to watch, entertaining, or humorous. They also listen and respond to advertisements that tell them about new products. A smaller percentage, but still a majority, of adults respond positively to advertisements that make them feel good about the product.[5]

ADVERTISING PLAN

In addition to a long-term planning commitment, advertising requires a significant financial investment. Therefore, market research in the form of a feasibility study should be done to determine if the expense of advertising will justify the income generated.

Although advertising is a creative process and must be consistent with the organization's objectives, position, image, and service benefits, advertising *requires* the use of professionals. It is an aspect of marketing that simply cannot be effectively performed in-house—with the possible exception of a small advertisement in the Yellow Pages. Before choosing an advertising agency, physical therapists should

- discuss their personal advertising philosophy and preferences
- study samples of work done for other clients
- find out what resources the agency uses (e.g., whether they are on site or contracted)
- determine the agency's perception of the clinic and its position in the marketplace
- learn what the agency expects from the clinic staff in terms of response time and meetings
- find out how the agency is organized
- determine who will work on what part of the project
- make sure that the agency's office hours correspond to their needs
- ask the agency about its guidelines for working on the clinic's account

Very large advertising agencies can be ruled out for most physical therapy clinics, because they rarely work with accounts involving less than $500,000 per year. Even small agencies look for clients with an annual advertising budget of approximately $50,000. Considering that service industries spend 3.5 percent of their gross income on advertising, an organization would require gross sales greater than one million dollars per year to undertake an advertising campaign in the $50,000 per year range. Smaller budgets may necessitate use of project-by-project contracts with an agency or free-lancer.[6] Therapists who are on the verge of committing themselves to the expense of advertising must be sure of what they are doing, why they are doing it, whom they are doing it for, and when they can reasonably expect a return on investment for their advertising dollars.

Staff members must work with the advertising agency to develop the clinic's marketing plan for the annual advertising mix. The advertising plan should include:

- goals
- market research
- advertising strategies
- evaluation.

Marketing goals can be coordinated with the organization's strategic plan. For example, if the organization plans to increase volume and revenue through a work hardening program, a congruent advertising goal may be to increase the target public's awareness of the program and stimulate use of the service. The market research would include an environmental analysis of demographic and attitudinal trends in potential users, competitors, gaps in the marketplace, and potential risks. Advertising strategies would be selected from among the various media. The program would be evaluated by pre- and post-testing of the target market's awareness level and by asking patients on the intake card how they learned of the service.

Designing the Advertisement

When working with an advertising agency, therapists should ensure that the following six questions are fully answered before the agency begins to design the advertisement:

1. What is the specific objective for the ad?
2. Who is the target customer?
3. What is the major benefit that must be emphasized in order to achieve the advertising objective?
4. What information supports that benefit?
5. What other benefits should be mentioned?
6. What outcome justifies the purchase of advertising?

Health care advertising is different from product advertising in that it advertises a service that is intangible; it cannot be seen, felt, touched, or experienced in any way prior to the use of the service. Advertising must, therefore, create a tangible experience for the audience in a memorable way. The following six guidelines will make an ad tangible, memorable, and trigger an audience response:

1. Offer a big benefit.
2. Make it easy to see and read.
3. Establish audience identity.
4. Attract by being new.
5. Be believable.
6. Stress what is unique.

Physical therapy advertising should always present a professional image that engenders trust and knowledge; it can be used to educate and inform the target market. An advertisement should not contain physical therapy–specific jargon that the audience may not understand, however. Typical words to avoid are *modality, neuromuscular re-education*, and Latin anatomical names for body parts. The hard-sell sales pitch often used in advertising bargain products is almost always a mistake in health care advertising because it cheapens the service.

Evaluating the Advertisement

Prior to accepting the advertisement from the agency for release, several persons who are not familiar with the service should be asked to review the proposed advertisement and answer the following four questions:

1. To whom is the advertisement directed?
2. What are the product benefits described in the advertisement?
3. What is the product image that the advertisement suggests?
4. How does the advertisement provide a response to take action?

If the answers to these questions match the organization's strategic plan, the advertisement may be accepted.

SYNDICATED ADVERTISING

A syndicated, or generic, advertisement is general enough to be sold for use by other clinics in other parts of the United States. The cost of syndicated advertising is 33 percent to 60 percent less than the cost of creating original advertisements. Although there has been significant criticism concerning the ability of a syndicated advertisement to address any population and fit into any marketing plan effectively, this type of advertising may not be all bad. If considered wisely, a syndicated advertising may fit well into a clinic's marketing mix. Its use is increasing in health care.

YELLOW PAGES ADVERTISING

No matter what other marketing tools a clinic uses, chances are that it advertises in the Yellow Pages. As consumers become more pro-active in their choice of health care professionals, they are becoming more and more likely to consult the Yellow Pages when they decide that they need a physical therapist.

The advertisement should be distinctive and, as always, address the needs of prospective patients. For example, if the clinic has extended evening and weekend hours and that is important to its clientele, the hours should be displayed prominently in the advertisement. A large advertisement may be worthwhile, as it will stand out among those of competitors. For patients who are already familiar with the clinic's services, the name, address, and telephone number should be listed not only in the Yellow Pages under Physical Therapists, but also in the business section of the white pages. For easy readability, it is worth purchasing boldface type.

Now that most communities have two or more available Yellow Pages, it is necessary to determine which ones are more widely distributed. The clinic will benefit from advertising more heavily in the Yellow Pages that are distributed more widely. If it is possible to determine the demographics of the population that receive the Yellow Pages, it will be possible to target the most expensive advertisements.

As with any marketing effort, it is essential to track the response rate. A question can be placed on the clinic's patient intake form that asks how the patient learned of the clinic. The receptionist can monitor and chart the results monthly.

LEGAL AND ETHICAL ISSUES

Advertisements that contain false, deceptive, or unfair representations are not legal. Care must be taken not to misrepresent quality or results, and to avoid guarantees of cures or relief of suffering. Any price discounting or free offers must be special events. Testimonials must not exaggerate the benefits that were derived from physical therapy.

Those who continue to have difficulty with the ethics of advertising or believe that advertising is something suspect, particularly in the health care field, should remember the old saying that ''if you add to the truth, you subtract from it.'' Clear, honest advertising campaigns inform the targeted public accurately about the services that they will receive. Without that information, people may have incorrect impressions of what physical therapy is able to offer them. Truthful, widespread advertising about physical therapy is advantageous and beneficial to both the consumer and the practitioner, because it gives the consumer more information with which to make health care decisions.

NOTES

1. L. Sachs, *Do-It-Yourself Marketing for the Professional Practice* (Englewood Cliffs, N.J.: Prentice-Hall, Inc., 1986).

2. W.J. Winston, ed., *Advertising Handbook for Health Care Services* (New York: The Haworth Press, Inc., 1986), 19.

3. Ibid., 11.

4. P.W. Burton and S.C. Purvis, *Which Ad Polled Best?* (Lincolnwood, Ill.: NTC Business Books, 1986), 6.

5. Winston, *Advertising Handbook for Health Care Services*, 33.

6. E. Kari, "Syndicated Health Care Advertising Increasing Despite Some Doubts about Its Effectiveness," *Modern Health Care* 17 (1987):84.

chapter 7

Competition

Webster defines competition as,

> 1: the act or process of competing: rivalry; 2: a contest between rivals; 3: the effort of two or more parties acting independently to secure the business of a third party by offering the most favorable terms; 4: act or demand by two or more organisms or kinds of organisms for some environmental resource in short supply.[1]

DEVELOPMENT OF COMPETITION IN HEALTH CARE

Much has been written recently on the topic of competition in health care. In the early 1980s, the federal government decided to attempt to reduce the rising costs of health care by encouraging competition among health care organizations. One of the steps that the government took was to provide tax incentives for alternate means of ensuring the health care of the population of the United States, such as health maintenance organizations and preferred provider organizations.

At the same time, Medicare began putting limits and caps on its expenditures. Private insurance companies followed suit and included limitations and caps on coverage in their policies. These actions reduced the pool of money to be used on health care expenditures in the United States and created a condition of "rivalry" among health care providers for available resources. Hospitals began to make efforts to offer more favorable terms and benefits to patients and physicians than did competing hospitals in the community. Major health care magazines started carrying articles on "competing to win" and other such topics.

Physical therapists were not immune to increasing competition in the health care arena. Physical therapy departments in hospitals were used to position the facilities as leaders in their communities because of their sports fitness and rehabilitation programs. The benefits of physical therapy were touted to the community as an example of a facility's differential advantage. Physical therapy departments also suffered as a result of the reduced reimbursement for all health care and increased competition. Budgets were slashed, departmental growth was often-times reduced, and expectations were increased. Pressure from management to increase their competitive advantage was felt in every department of successful health care organizations in the 1980s.

Several strategies for managing competition in the health care arena were developed. A common strategy was to take the militaristic viewpoint. This approach emphasizes winning and surviving under conditions in which competitors are viewed as the enemy. The focus is on the competitors' strengths and weaknesses, and the goal is to win by selecting offensive or defensive strategies. A second strategy to deal with competition is to monitor the competitive market share in the community, as well as competitive marketing strategies. This information can be used as a stimulus and a challenge to improve an organization. The focus of the first competitive strategy is on the competitor. The focus of the second is on the organization's relationship with the consumer.

Although it is valuable to understand the military approach to coping with competition in health care, it is more effective in the long run for an organization to focus on its own program, to improve its own product, and to increase its market share through excellence rather than through a short-term fix, such as stealing patients from the competitor. More recent literature notes that health care facilities are "in business to serve a purpose and carry out a mission, not to survive or beat out their competitors."[2] Treating the community as a battleground for various health care providers may be a necessity in order to react to competitive pressures, in the short-term, but health care organizations that do not lose their own consumer focus in these battles will win the war by recognizing that the primary goal is providing a service to the community.

BENEFITS OF COMPETITION

Competition can be beneficial if it stimulates an organization to change, to analyze its own position in the marketplace, and to undertake strategic planning efforts. It can motivate management to monitor, assess, and change current performance standards constantly to promote excellence. When competition is viewed as a devil's advocate to bring out the best in everyone, it can be a healthy and useful force in the marketplace.

As Davidson stated, "the healthy competitor has the edge, in part, because he has much less competitive stress than the traditional competitor has, giving him much more energy for the task at hand!"[3] Davidson noted that, in competing, the healthy competitor must be innovative and creative, rather than imitating, comparing, and confirming with the competition. As physical therapists continue to cope with rising competition for the health care dollar, they should look at their competitors as devil's advocates, rather than rivals, and plan their strategies based on innovation and creativity, rather than on imitation and comparison.

ANALYSIS OF THE COMPETITION

An organization rarely stands alone in its efforts to serve a given customer market. Its efforts to build an efficient marketing system to serve that market are matched by similar efforts on the part of others. The competitive environment includes not only other physical therapy clinics, but also other means of achieving physical therapy goals. Thus, the typical consumer has a number of choices when faced with such conditions as functional deficits, pain due to musculoskeletal dysfunction, postural problems, spinal malalignment, and deconditioning.

Consumer Choices

The consumer with a problem that physical therapy could address successfully has at least four choices. The individual may choose not to pay for health care to solve the problem, but to try self-medication through over-the-counter drugs, to design an exercise program by reading the literature, or simply to ask friends or relatives for advice. The consumer's second choice is to pay for health care. The consumer who has made this decision may seek medical care or nonmedical care (e.g., from an alternative health care practitioner, such as a massage therapist). The third consumer choice falls within the medical model; the consumer may go to a physical therapist or to a physician for medication or for surgery. The fourth and final choice must be made by the consumer who decides to undergo physical therapy as a method of solving the physical problem; that person must then choose among physical therapy services. When therapists assess their competition, they must be sure to include all four levels of competition.

The important goal of a competitive strategy is to increase the clinic's market share. This increase does not necessarily need to come from the current market share of other physical therapy services. The strategic approach may be to increase total market share by marketing to a consumer group that has not previously used physical therapy to solve its musculoskeletal problems.

Marketing Strategies for All Levels

A comprehensive marketing strategy plan addresses all four levels of competitors and includes strategies to target each of these four levels. The current and future competitive marketing strategies directed to each of the four levels of competitors should be profiled (Exhibit 7-1). The percentage of marketing efforts that went into these various physical therapy competitors last year should be determined, and plans made to distribute marketing strategies among all four competitors next year. Following are strategies that can be used for each of the four consumer positions:

- consumers who choose not to pay for care
  1. Give lectures to community groups.
  2. Attend health fairs.
  3. Encourage word-of-mouth promotions from patients.
  4. Request testimonial advertising.
  5. Undertake multiple exposure marketing.
- consumers who choose nontraditional medicine
  1. Give lectures to community groups.
  2. Attend health fairs.
  3. Encourage word-of-mouth promotions from patients.
  4. Request testimonial advertising.
  5. Undertake multiple exposure marketing.
  6. Advertise physical therapy benefits in newspapers and magazines targeted to this audience.
  7. Make sales calls to nontraditional practitioners to discuss when referrals are appropriate.
- consumers who choose prescription medication or surgery
  1. Make sales calls to physicians.
  2. Distribute brochures.
  3. Send out newsletters.
  4. Perform telecommunications marketing.
  5. Encourage word-of-mouth promotion from patients.
- consumers who choose physical therapy
  1. Develop and promote differential advantage.
  2. Position the clinic with benefits expected by consumers.
  3. Stay visible and prominent with referral sources.
  4. Develop relationships with payors.

In developing the marketing plan, the therapists should take into account the fact that the consumer who has already chosen to receive physical therapy is the most likely to seek care at their clinic. The consumer who chooses not to pay for care will be the most difficult to reach and will require the most extensive marketing efforts. Because the traditional medical marketplace is not currently reaching this consumer either, however, creating a marketing method to reach this particular consumer may be extremely profitable.

Exhibit 7-1 Competitive Marketing Plan

Physical Therapy Competitor Level	Percent of Market Plan Last Year	Percent of Market Plan Next Year
1. Consumer who chooses not to pay for care	_____	_____
2. Consumer who chooses nontraditional medicine	_____	_____
3. Consumer who chooses prescription medication or surgery	_____	_____
4. Consumer who chooses physical therapy	_____	_____

ASSESSMENT OF COMPETITORS

Once the competitors have been identified, the competitors' services should be examined to determine if they differ from the clinic's services. One way to evaluate a competitor's services is to perform a facility assessment (see Chapter 3). If there are gaps in the staff's knowledge of a competitor's facility, it may be necessary to do some research. The first step is simply to call the facility and ask. If there are still gaps in the information, a therapist may visit the facility and ask for a tour through the clinic. Alternatively, a therapist may ask colleagues for information about the competitors.

The next step is to compare the clinic's strengths with the competition's weaknesses in terms of what the consumer wants from a physical therapy clinic. The clinic's differential advantage is established on the basis of its strengths.

The competitors' market shares can often be determined by calling each clinic in the community and asking what its volume was in the preceding year and comparing the various volumes by percentage to the total physical therapy volume in the community. This market share analysis should be performed at least annually to determine the effectiveness of the clinic's marketing efforts and to track its share of the market in comparison to the competitors' shares. It is important to keep records of the total physical therapy market volume in the community over time to determine if the market for physical therapy is increasing, decreasing, or staying the same and to calculate the percentage of any change.

The clinic staff should determine if the various competitors have any striking features that help them attract clients. The strengths and weaknesses of competitors should be assessed. The marketing strategies that are used by the competitors and the way in which they are positioning themselves in the marketplace should be examined. An effort should be made to determine what the competitors' goals and assumptions are for increasing their share of the marketplace.

It is helpful to know a competitor's costs of doing business, particularly if these costs vary or differ from the clinic's costs. For example, a physical therapy department located in a hospital may need to share overhead costs with the rest of the hospital, including non–revenue-producing departments (e.g., nursing). The physical therapy clinic that is located in a high rent district obviously has higher costs than does the physical therapy clinic located in other areas. The location of each competitor should be evaluated not only in terms of cost of space rental or purchase, but also in terms of accessibility to public transportation and parking, proximity to other health care facilities, and location in business community versus residential community. In sum, a therapist should ask the following questions when analyzing competitors:

- Who are the competitors?
- Do the competitors' services differ from yours?
- What is the competitors' share of the market?
- Do the competitors have any striking features that help them attract clients?
- What are the competitors' strengths and weaknesses?
- What are the competitors' marketing strategies?
- What are the competitors' goals and assumptions?
- What are the competitors' costs?
- What are the features of the competitors' location?

Competitor information can be gathered without resorting to corporate espionage. In general, therapists should always stay open to information concerning their competitors. Staff members should monitor and record any information that they receive concerning the competition. For example, patients who have been to competitors often make comments, both positive and negative.

Information specifically for the competitor analysis can be gathered through direct conversations and networking. The best way to obtain information about competitors is to attend professional meetings and talk to them. A therapist should not hesitate to call a competitor and ask questions. A more "covert" way to gather information about competitors is to shop the facility as a prospective user, either by telephone or in person.[4] It is surprising how much information a switchboard operator or receptionist will provide without question. Examination of the brochures and marketing tools used by competitors also helps to reveal their marketing position.

STRATEGIES FOR DEALING WITH COMPETITION

There are four basic approaches to take in dealing with the competition: (1) the win-lose approach, (2) the win-win approach, (3) the imitation approach, and

Exhibit 7-2 Strategies for Dealing with Competition

1. Create win-loose situation over the competition
2. Create win-win situation with the competition
3. Imitate the competition
4. Ignore the competition

(4) the approach that simply ignores the competition (Exhibit 7-2). Although there are circumstances in which each approach is appropriate, the win-win approach is recommended as the most likely to succeed within the health care community.

Win-Lose Approach

Creating a win-lose situation with the competition may be the strategy of choice in a market that has very little room for growth. In order for one organization to grow, another organization must become smaller. In following this strategy, it is essential to recognize the reality that competition cannot be overrun in a short period of time. A reputation must develop gradually. Rational, honest marketing strategies should be used to increase market share.

Win-Win Approach

Creating a win-win situation with the competition is the best strategy to follow, if at all possible. "Partnership provides a much stronger basis for motivating key stakeholders toward the goal of improving the community's health."[5] A win-win situation with the competition is by far the most productive competitive strategy, for it makes a colleague rather than an enemy of the competition.

A win-win situation requires cooperation among competitors. There are three ways for competitors to cooperate with each other: bargaining, co-optation, and coalition. Cooperating with a competitor means that both parties are willing to work toward mutual goals through a predetermined degree of involvement with each other.

Bargaining is a negotiated effort; the future behavior of both parties is negotiated to a satisfactory conclusion. For example, two private practice physical therapy clinics that are located in close proximity to one another may negotiate an agreement in which one clinic agrees to specialize in geriatrics while the other clinic agrees to specialize in sports medicine. Both parties win in this situation, and neither party is trying to capture the other's market share.

Co-optation occurs when two organizations agree in some way to become a part of each other. If a hospital's physical therapy outpatient department perceives that the local private practice physical therapist is pulling a large market share from the hospital, for example, it may offer the private practice physical therapist a contract to provide physical therapy services in the hospital. By accepting the contract, the private practice physical therapist is co-opted with the hospital to provide those services. In this way, both parties have won.

A coalition between competing organizations combines services for a common purpose beneficial to all. A number of coalitions of private practitioners have been formed around the United States for the purpose of negotiating with insurance companies, making group purchases, and performing marketing activities.

Imitation

The strategy of imitating the competitor is sometimes appropriate. A product leader incurs many costs involving market research, product development, implementation, and marketing. Imitating the competitor sometimes allows a clinic to piggyback on the competitor's costly research and marketing efforts. The expenses incurred as the second entry in the marketplace are much less than those of the first entry. Therefore, the imitator can invest in other aspects of the product, such as making it better. The weakness of the strategy is that it does not define the organization as a product leader.

Ignoring the Competition

It is never a good strategy to ignore the competition, because a clinic that adopts this policy is likely to lose at least a portion of its market share to stronger competitive practices. As the health care dollar shrinks through reduced insurance reimbursement, competition becomes a reality in health care; physical therapy is not immune to this competition. The physical therapist has many choices in assessing, managing, and interacting with the competition. It is always best to have as much information as possible about competitors, their strengths and weaknesses, their marketing strategies, their differential advantage, and the benefits that they promote to the public.

NOTES

1. *Webster's Ninth New Collegiate Dictionary* (Springfield, Mass.: Merriam-Webster, Inc., 1984).
2. R.S. MacStravic, "Warfare or Partnership: Which Way for Health Care?" *Health Care Management Review* (1990):37–45.

3. J. Davidson, ''Competing to Win: Healthy Stress-free Competition,'' *Physical Therapy Today* 12 (1989).

4. Mystery Shopper, *Marketing News,* June 5, 1987.

5. MacStravic, ''Warfare or Partnership.''

Epilogue

Incorporating a marketing approach into the administrative and clinical aspects of a physical therapy service can be easy, enjoyable, rewarding, and profitable. The dynamic use of the organization's differential advantage, positioning, target markets, and hierarchy of effects focuses all business activities toward the organization's mission and purpose.

Marketing is the communication between the organization and its target markets. Within a comprehensive marketing program, this communication not only is focused and controlled, but also pervades both external promotions and internal staff attitudes. Additionally, the organization's target markets receive a unified, consistent message that helps break through the information clutter of today's society. Decision making for the consumer and other target markets is simplified and clarified, so informed and appropriate clients are directed toward the organization. In this way, the marketing function assists employees and clients in their communications, thereby increasing the satisfaction of both groups. Increased employee satisfaction reduces turnover and enhances a positive clinic environment. When all employees realize that they are part of the marketing team, they become invested as important contributors to the organization's success. Increased customer satisfaction engenders repeat business and positive word-of-mouth promotions—the final goal of most marketing efforts.

Index

Page numbers in *italics* denote exhibits; page numbers followed by a "t" denote tables.

DATE DUE

OCT 1 1 1999			
OCT 2 5 1999			
APR 0 2 2000			